John T. Pardeck, PhD

Using Books in Clinical Social Work Practice
A Guide to Bibliotherapy

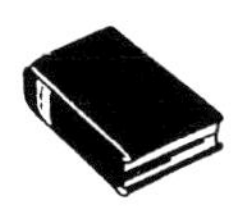

Pre-publication
REVIEWS,
COMMENTARIES,
EVALUATIONS . . .

"*Using Books in Clinical Social Work Practice: A Guide to Bibliotherapy* is theoretically sound, well researched, clearly organized, and easy to follow, with many relevant applications discussed, and ends with a great annotated bibliography. In-depth treatment is given to several social problems that are often the focus of clinical interventions. Furthermore, a thorough review of both the benefits and shortcomings of bibliotherapy is provided. In the end, a complete program of bibliography is outlined."

John W. Murphy, PhD
Professor of Sociology,
University of Miami,
Coral Gables, FL

More pre-publication
REVIEWS, COMMENTARIES, EVALUATIONS . . .

"Social work practitioners and others who engage in helping relationships with others will find *Using Books in Clinical Social Work Practice: A Guide to Bibliotherapy* by John T. Pardeck informative, well-written, and in general a great resource. In an accessible and interesting style, Pardeck outlines the history and theoretical basis of bibliotherapy as well as the more practical skills needed by therapists and counselors who choose this mode of intervention. This book includes an impressive review of the research on bibliotherapy. Furthermore, detailed therapy and counseling techniques are provided. One chapter is designed as an annotated bibliography of fiction and nonfiction readings that could be utilized in bibliotherapy. This book is an invaluable reference for both novice and experienced practitioners who want to develop bibliotherapeutic techniques."

Karen A. Callaghan, PhD
Associate Professor and Chair,
Department of Sociology
and Criminology,
Barry University,
Miami Shores, FL

"The material in this book is well conceived within the context of the empirical evidence available on the effectiveness of bibliotherapy. Moreover, the subject warrants this long-overdue book-length treatment at a time when resources for human services are limited and/or eliminated completely. This book can provide clinicians with a framework for expediently addressing the problems of many individuals in society, such as the grief a child experiences in losing a parent to divorce or death.

Given that the book is well organized, cogent, and timely, it will be of interest to professionals and laypersons alike. Bravo to Pardeck for giving us this practical, functional guide to using books in our work with clients of all ages."

Martha Markward, PhD
School of Social Work,
University of Georgia,
Athens, GA

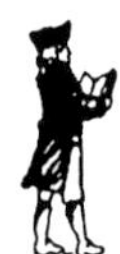

The Haworth Press, Inc.

NOTES FOR PROFESSIONAL LIBRARIANS AND LIBRARY USERS

This is an original book title published by The Haworth Press, Inc. Unless otherwise noted in specific chapters with attribution, materials in this book have not been previously published elsewhere in any format or language.

CONSERVATION AND PRESERVATION NOTES

All books published by The Haworth Press, Inc. and its imprints are printed on certified ph neutral, acid free book grade paper. This paper meets the minimum requirements of American National Standard for Information Sciences–Permanence of Paper for Printed Material, ANSI Z39.48-1984.

Using Books in Clinical Social Work Practice
A Guide to Bibliotherapy

THE HAWORTH PRESS

New, Recent, and Forthcoming Titles of Related Interest

Gerontological Social Work Supervision by Ann Burack-Weiss and Frances Coyle Brennan

Group Work: Skills and Strategies for Effective Interventions by Sondra Brandler and Camille P. Roman

If a Partner Has AIDS: Guide to Clinical Intervention for Relationships in Crisis by R. Dennis Shelby

Elements of the Helping Process: A Guide for Clinicians by Raymond Fox

Clinical Social Work Supervision, Second Edition by Carlton E. Munson

Intervention Research: Design and Development for the Human Services edited by Jack Rothman and Edwin J. Thomas

Forensic Social Work: Legal Aspects of Professional Practice by Robert L. Barker and Douglas M. Branson

Now Dare Everything: Tales of HIV-Related Psychotherapy by Steven F. Dansky

The Black Elderly: Satisfaction and Quality of Later Life by Marguerite M. Coke and James A. Twaite

Building on Women's Strengths: A Social Work Agenda for the Twenty-First Century by Liane V. Davis

Family Beyond Family: The Surrogate Parent in Schools and Other Community Agencies by Sanford Weinstein

The Cross-Cultural Practice of Clinical Case Management in Mental Health edited by Peter Manoleas

Environmental Practice in the Human Services: Integration of Micro and Macro Roles, Skills, and Contexts by Bernard Neugeboren

Basic Social Policy and Planning: Strategies and Practice Methods by Hobart A. Burch

Fundamentals of Cognitive-Behavior Therapy: From Both Sides of the Desk by Bill Borcherdt

Social Work Intervention in an Economic Crisis: The River Communities Project by Martha Baum and Pamela Twiss

The Relational Systems Model for Family Therapy: Living in the Four Realities by Donald R. Bardill

Feminist Theories and Social Work: Approaches and Applications by Christine Flynn Saulnier

Social Work Approaches to Conflict Resolution: Making Fighting Obsolete by Benyamin Chetkow-Yanoov

Principles of Social Work Practice: A Generic Practice Approach by Molly R. Hancock

Nobody's Children: Orphans of the HIV Epidemic by Steven F. Dansky

Social Work in Health Settings: Practice in Context, Second Edition by Toba Schwaber Kerson and Associates

Critical Social Welfare Issues: Tools for Social Work and Health Care Professionals edited by Arthur J. Katz, Abraham Lurie, and Carlos Vidal

Social Work Practice: A Systems Approach, Second Edition by Benyamin Chetkow-Yanoov

Using Books in Clinical Social Work Practice

A Guide to Bibliotherapy

John T. Pardeck, PhD

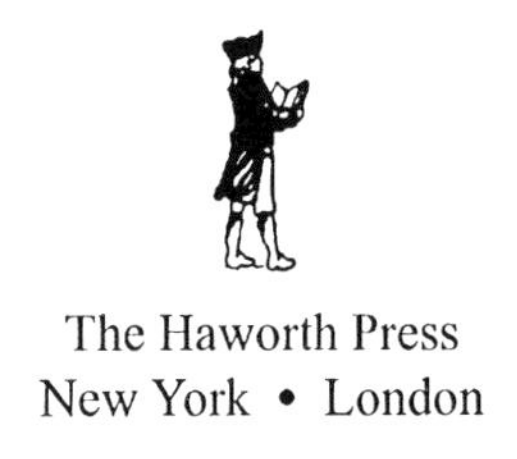

The Haworth Press
New York • London

The Haworth Press, Inc., 10 Alice Street, Binghamton, NY 13904-1580

Cover design by Monica L. Seifert.

Library of Congress Cataloging-in-Publication Data

Pardeck, John T.
Using books in clinical social work practice : a guide to bibliotherapy / John T. Pardeck.
p. cm.
Includes bibliographical references (p.) and index.
ISBN 0-7890-0430-5 (alk. paper).
1. Bibliotherapy. 2. Psychiatric social work. I. Title.
RC489.B48P37 1997
615.8'516–dc21 97-30713
CIP

To Jean A. Pardeck, Jonathan T. Pardeck,
and James K. Pardeck, my family

ABOUT THE AUTHOR

John T. Pardeck, PhD, is Professor of Social Work in the School of Social Work at Southeast Missouri State University. He is a member of the Academy of Certified Social Workers (ACSW) and a Licensed Clinical Social Worker (LCSW) in the state of Missouri. Dr. Pardeck has published over 100 articles in academic and professional journals, as well as several books. His most recent books include *Computers in Human Services: An Overview for Clinical and Welfare Services* (1990), *The Computerization of Human Services Agencies: A Critical Appraisal* (1991), *Issues in Social Work: A Critical Analysis* with Roland G. Meinert and William P. Sullivan (1994), and *Social Work Practice: An Ecological Approach* (1996).

CONTENTS

Foreword

The literature in the helping professions, in particular books and journal articles on social work, have dealt with the utility of bibliotherapy in clinical practice in a minimal and peripheral fashion. Thus, Professor Pardeck's most recent effort in this area makes a contribution to the bibliotherapeutic literature by providing social work clinicians with information about not only the value of the approach itself, but specific guidelines for its application in professional practice.

The appearance of this book is quite timely given the recent and dramatic developments that have taken place in the health and human service fields. For example, in the health field, the rapid rise of managed care with its emphasis on alternative forms of therapy, cost containment, and short-term treatment dictates that professional social workers become conversant with the applicability of variable treatment options. Bibliotherapy is one of the options that has relevance to the treatment directions now underway in the managed care field. As Pardeck points out, bibliotherapy may be selected as the primary treatment focus or an ancillary to it with careful thought and judgment. This book provides the clinical practitioner with the required information to exercise that judgment.

The underlying logic and plan by which Pardeck presents material about bibliotherapy touches all the conceptual and practical bases. The serious reader of this book will come away with a better understanding of the history of bibliotherapy; the research studies that have shed light on it; the strengths and weaknesses of the approach; guidelines for its use in practice; and suggestions about fiction and nonfiction readings that apply to several client problem areas. Both experienced clinicians and clinicians in training will find the last section of the book of direct value to practice. Pardeck identifies over 300 books that have applicability to several clinical topics. Each book is followed by an annotated critical commentary to assist in making a decision about its use in specific clinical therapeutic situations.

Many of the over 530 accredited social work education programs at both the baccalaureate and master's levels have an emphasis on preparing professional social workers for clinical practice. The conventional wisdom of many program directors and clinical instructors is to present students with in-depth information about the currently popular theoretical approaches to treatment that appear in the literature. Unfortunately, bibliotherapy has not been visible within this written genre. Pardeck's book is a welcome addition to the clinical treatment literature and provides educational programs with a solid and well-researched guide to the many values of the bibliotherapeutic alternative.

Clinicians wedded to a specific theoretical or ideological approach to treatment will also find value in Pardeck's discussion of bibliotherapy and the practical guidelines for applying it in practice. The bibliotherapeutic guidelines he presents cut across fields of practice and theoretical positions since they are problem-focused. It applies, therefore, to social work practice in general regardless of one's therapeutic orientation, and thus is a contribution to the entire field of clinical practice and not just a segment of it.

Roland G. Meinert, PhD
President, Missouri Association for Social Welfare

Preface

PURPOSE

The purpose of this book is to provide clinical social workers with books that can be used to treat various clinical problems. The approach offered for using books in clinical intervention is bibliotherapy. Bibliotherapy is an emerging clinical technique that has been found useful for treating various clinical problems. Chapter 1 offers an introduction to the bibliotherapeutic approach, explains who uses it in practice, and gives a detailed review of the research literature on the topic of bibliotherapy.

Chapter 2 presents the clinical applications of bibliotherapy. This chapter covers utilizing bibliotherapy with fiction and nonfiction books. Strategies are offered for using bibliotherapy with individuals and groups.

Chapter 3 provides a brief overview of the clinical topics covered in the book. These include divorce and remarriage, dysfunctional families, parenting, self-development, serious illness, and substance abuse related disorders. Chapter 4 offers useful books for treating problems related to the issues covered in Chapter 3. In Chapter 4, there are over 300 annotated books presented that deal with these potential problem areas. Titles are offered for both children and adults.

COVERAGE AND SCOPE

The majority of books annotated in this work were published in the mid-1980s to the present; a limited number of the books are from earlier time periods. The general criteria used for selecting a book were that:

1. The book had to focus on one or more of the clinical topics covered in the work.
2. The book had to offer useful content on the problem area covered.
3. The book had to be clearly appropriate to the implementation of the bibliotherapeutic process.

Each book has an Interest Level (IL) indicated by age. If the Interest Level of the book is over eighteen years of age, the IL is followed by the word Adult. The reader will be able to gain insight into the book's content through the work's annotation; the annotation also provides enough information to allow the reader to judge if a work is fiction or nonfiction.

ENTRIES

The annotated entries included are arranged in alphabetical order under each topic area by the author's last name. Many of the annotated works focus on more than one clinical problem. However, the primary clinical problem covered in a given work determined the problem area under which it was included. For example, a book on marriage and divorce may include some content on dysfunctional families. If the primary focus is on marriage and divorce, however, the book was placed in that topic area.

INDEXES

The Author Index is a guide to the authors who wrote the books annotated in each problem area. The Title Index helps the reader locate a particular title. The numbers following the authors and titles in these two indexes refer to the book's main entry numbers within each of the problem areas in Chapter 4. A Subject Index allows the reader to refer to specific subjects covered in the annotated entries. Like the two other indexes, the Subject Index refers the reader to the appropriate number in Chapter 4.

Acknowledgments

The author appreciates the encouragement of Jean Pardeck, Ruth Pardeck, Lois Musick, and Burl Musick. They all provided help during the preparation of this book.

Chapter 1

An Introduction to Bibliotherapy

Books have been used as a therapeutic tool since ancient times. In ancient Greece, for example, the door of a library at Thebes bore the inscription, "The Healing Place of the Soul." During the nineteenth century in the United States, the *McGuffey Reader* and *The New England Primer* were used as primary teaching tools as well as resources for building character and developing positive values in students.

One of the earliest individuals to use reading as a tool for helping individuals deal with mental health problems was Dr. William C. Menninger. Dr. Menninger was also interested in how the layperson might use popular literature in the areas of psychiatry and psychology. He found that books such as *The Human Mind,* written by his brother Karl A. Menninger (1945), were widely used by many laypersons and mental health professionals as tools for dealing with mental health problems. Given the positive reaction to *The Human Mind,* the Menningers became advocates of using bibliotherapy in the therapeutic process. In fact, the interest the Menningers showed in self-help books led to many mental hospitals offering bibliotherapy as a program of treatment (Starker, 1986). However, the Menningers strongly advised against prescribing mental health literature to psychotic individuals, those with anxiety states or obsessional neuroses, and those in psychoanalysis. They deemed bibliotherapy as an appropriate treatment for mild neuroses, alcoholism, for relatives of patients, and for parents who needed help in child guidance (Starker, 1988).

Since the Menningers's endorsement of self-help books as a mental health tool, increasing numbers of practitioners have begun using this emerging technology in treatment. During the 1960s and

1970s, numerous self-help books were published; at present, millions of Americans use self-help books and other kinds of written materials for dealing with problems ranging from advice on diets to personal growth.

Bibliotherapy has been known by several names, including bibliocounseling, bibliopsychology, biblioeducation, biblioguidance, library therapeutics, biblioprophylaxis, tutorial group therapy, and literatherapy (Rubin, 1978). *Webster's New Collegiate Dictionary* (1981, p. 25) defines bibliotherapy as "guidance in the solution of personal problems through directed reading." Berry (1978, p. 185) defines "bibliotherapy as a family of techniques for structuring an interaction between a facilitator and a participant . . . based on their mutual sharing of literature." Regardless of how one defines it, over the last several decades bibliotherapy has been used by many professionals including counselors, psychologist, psychiatrists, and educators. Social workers have only recently begun to use bibliotherapy in clinical practice (Pardeck and Pardeck, 1983, 1987, 1989). In fact, Barker's (1995) *Dictionary of Social Work* includes a comprehensive definition for bibliotherapy:

> The use of literature and poetry in the treatment of people with emotional problems or mental illness. Bibliotherapy is often used in social group work and group therapy and is reported to be effective with people of all ages, with people in institutions as well as outpatients, and with healthy people who wish to share literature as a means of personal growth and development. (p. 35)

Even though social workers have only recently begun to use bibliotherapy as a clinical tool, as with other professionals, social workers have only minimal preparation in the use of this emerging treatment technique (Rubin, 1978).

RESEARCH ON BIBLIOTHERAPY

Fiction and nonfiction books can be used when treating clients with bibliotherapy. Even though evidence suggests fiction can be a useful therapeutic tool, the research findings strongly suggest behavioral- and cognitive-based reading materials in the form of nonfiction self-help books have the greatest empirical support (Pardeck, 1993).

During the 1980s, fourteen studies were conducted on the effects of bibliotherapy as a tool for changing behavior through self-help books. Of these studies, only three suggest bibliotherapy is not effective. Four studies report bibliotherapy can be a useful tool for changing inappropriate behaviors of adolescents (Harbaugh, 1984; Miller, 1982; Swantic, 1986; Frankel and Merbaun, 1982). Pezzot-Pearce, LeBow, and Pearce (1982) reported bibliotherapy in the form of self-help books can be used as a successful tool for reducing weight. Bailey (1982) found that reading a self-help manual effectively treated insomnia. Rucker (1983) and Cuevas (1984) report that behaviorally based self-help books effectively treated obesity and chronic headaches. Of three studies using comparison treatment groups, one found self-help books effective in changing children's behavior (Klingman, 1985), another found them useful in improving conversation skills (Black, 1981), and a third discovered self-help books helped clients lose weight (Black and Threlfall, 1986). Conner (1981) reported that self-help books did not improve interpersonal skills. Galliford (1982) found no evidence for their effectiveness in weight control. Giles (1986) concluded that reading stories describing reinforcement contingencies did not shape the immediate behavior of clinically disturbed children.

More recent research in the 1990s continues to support the effectiveness of self-help books in clinical practice. Four studies found self-help books useful for treating health-related problems. Starker (1992a, 1992b, 1994) in three studies found that self-help books improved clients' attitudes toward health problems and treatment, provided therapeutic comfort, and lowered stress levels in clients receiving medical health-related services. Matthews and Lonsdale (1992) found that children who were hospitalized benefited from self-help books.

In the area of mental health, Gould, Clum, and Shapiro (1995) concluded in their research that self-help books can effectively help treat clients suffering from agoraphobia. Lesser (1991) found self-help reading as a useful adjunct for treating panic disorders. Ellis (1993) and Halliday (1991) concluded in their respective studies that self-help books enabled clients to make profound personality changes. Ogles, Lambert, and Craig (1991) found self-help reading useful as a tool for helping clients deal with loss related to marital breakdown. Long, Rickert, and Ashcraft (1993) concluded that self-help materials are an excellent adjunct for treating attention deficit disorders in children. Only two studies reported that self-help books offered limited success for treating clinical problems. Aldridge and Clayton (1990) and Forest (1991) concluded from their research that self-help reading materials were not particularly helpful as therapeutic tools. Finally, research not focusing on treatment outcome but rather on the use of self-help books by professionals found female therapists more often recommended self-help reading materials to their clients compared to male therapists (Marx et al., 1992).

Given the fact that most studies in the 1980s and 1990s reported self-help books were effective in treatment, these findings suggest practitioners can use self-help books with some confidence in therapy. However, the following review of the literature focusing on the use of fiction in treatment suggests that the research evidence is not as great for this form of bibliotherapy.

Fiction, poetry, or inspirational readings have limited empirical support as bibliotherapeutic treatment mediums. This may be the case because behavioral and cognitive oriented self-help books are more amenable to empirical scrutiny (Pardeck, 1993).

During the 1980s, a number of studies analyzed the effect that fiction and other related reading materials had on changing the self-concepts of individuals. Bohlmann (1986), Ray (1983), and Taylor (1982) all reported success in using fiction in bibliotherapy treatment for improving the self-concepts of client. However, DeFrances and colleagues (1982) and Shafron (1983) found no support for improving self-concept through fiction books.

Other studies report mixed results on the effectiveness of fiction in treatment. Ford, Bashford, and DeWitt (1984) discovered limited support for its effectiveness in marital counseling. Libman and colleagues (1984) found some success in using fiction in family counseling for sexual dysfunction. Dodge, Glasgow, and O'Neill's (1982) research concludes that fiction is effective in treating sexual dysfunction. Finally, Morris-Vann (1983) and Sadler (1982) reported fiction and other non-behavioral-oriented self-help readings were effective in improving emotional adjustment of clients.

More recent studies from the 1990s focusing on the use of fiction in bibliotherapeutic treatment report a number of positive treatment outcomes. Cohen (1993) concluded, in a study focusing on adults, that the reading of literature reduced stress levels in clients. Similar findings were reported by Gaffney (1993). Coleman and Ganong (1990) found juvenile fiction to be a very useful tool for helping therapists work with children of stepfamilies. The emerging need to treat the emotional problems of homeless children was the focus of a study by Farkas and Yorker (1993). This research reports that fiction books were effective for working with homeless children. Research by Lanza (1996) reports that fiction books can promote emotional catharsis, active problem solving, and insight into problems. Even with the many positive studies conducted thus far in the 1990s focusing on the effectiveness of literature in treatment, Pardeck and Markward (1995) concluded that is is critical to continue to conduct research on the efficacy of bibliotherapy.

PURPOSE AND GOALS

The purposes of bibliotherapy include the following: (1) to provide information, (2) to provide insight, (3) to stimulate discussion about problems, (4) to communicate new values and attitudes, (5) to create awareness that others have similar problems, (6) to provide solutions to problems, and (7) to provide realistic solutions to problems (Baruth and Burggraf, 1984; Orton, 1997).

Various kinds of information can be conveyed through assigned and shared reading. Through bibliotherapy new facts can be discovered, different ways to approach problems can be understood, and alternative ways of thinking about and solving problems may be presented (Orton, 1997). These functions of bibliotherapy are particularly helpful to clients confronted with various kinds of clinical problems, since most clients have limited prior knowledge or personal experience with the problems confronting them.

Insight, or self-awareness, is another important goal of bibliotherapy (Santrock, Minnett, and Campbell, 1994). When practitioners use fiction in bibliotherapy, for example, clients can read about a character facing a problem similar to their own, they my identify with the character, and in so doing gain some awareness and insight into their own motivations, thoughts, and feelings (Griffin, 1984). By reading about a character's conflicts and emotional reactions, a client can gain insight into a presenting problem (Pardeck, 1991a).

Bibliotherapy can be a novel technique for stimulating discussion about a problem which otherwise may not be discussed because of fear, guilt, or shame. With the help of the therapist, reading can also be used as a medium to help clients verbalize feelings about a confronting problem (Bernstein, 1989).

Bibliotherapy has been found useful for changing attitudes and values. Standley and Standley (1970), and Shechtman (1994) found bibliotherapy had a positive impact on changing attitudes of majority group members toward minority populations. Doll and Doll (1997) also reported the positive impact that bibliotherapy had on changing attitudes and values. Given these findings, bibliotherapy can be used as a helpful technique particularly in educational settings for changing attitudes and values of individuals (Pardeck, 1993).

Finally, bibliotherapy can be a useful tool for helping clients confront and change presenting problems by reading about how others who have done so successfully. For example, an individual with a physical disability can read about a character who has successfully dealt with a similar disability. A person with a disability may learn that many others have faced the same problem, had similar feelings of inadequacy, and yet were able to develop self-realization about their disability (Pardeck and Pardeck, 1984).

VALUES OF BIBLIOTHERAPY

Practitioners who work with clients experiencing problems see great value in bibliotherapy. In particular, therapists can help clients gain insight into problems, provide them with techniques for relaxation and diversion, create a medium through which they can discuss problems, help clients focus outside themselves, and create an environment in which they can objectively discuss a situation in a book and apply it to their own situations (Pardeck, 1991a).

Even though practitioners have found bibliotherapy to be an effective treatment tool for a number of clinical problems, critics of the bibliotherapeutic technique claim it is far from an exact science. What must be noted, however, is virtually all of the helping therapies have limited scientific support; bibliotherapy is no exception (Pardeck, 1993). However, bibliotherapy may be more complex than other current therapies in that the therapist must be skilled in selecting literature and/or self-help books that parallel the problems facing a client as well as knowing how to use these materials as therapeutic mediums (Warner, 1991). If a practitioner can do this successfully, bibliotherapy can prove to be a very helpful treatment approach.

Bibliotherapy can also be useful for helping clients in their interpersonal relationships. For example, if a client is having problems with peer or family relationships, bibliotherapy can help in developing tolerance and understanding of others, creating acceptance of others, and formulating a more objective and rational approach to human problems. After reading about how other families work, a client faced with family problems can see that he or she has problems similar to others and that solutions are available. In turn, a client having problems with peers can gain insight into the complexities of peer relationships through reading books about other peer situations. This important insight can lead to solutions for the client with the assistance of the therapist (Pardeck, 1991a).

Finally, bibliotherapy may be seen as a preventive tool. For example, a rebellious adolescent may gain insight through reading about his or her behavior and find solutions to preventing future problems. A client might read about a developmental crisis and find solutions for dealing with it. Adolescents often have many concerns about human sexuality; books can be a useful tool for dealing with this critical developmental issue. In essence, books may be the only way that a client may see that he or she is not alone with a problem.

PRINCIPLES OF BIBLIOTHERAPY

Pardeck (1991b) and Rubin (1978) outline the major principles of bibliotherapy as follows:

1. The practitioner should use books with which he or she is familiar.
2. The therapist should be conscious of the length of the book. Complex books with extraneous details and situations should be avoided.
3. The client's problem must be considered; the book should be applicable to the problem facing the client.
4. The client's reading ability must be known and must guide the choice of books used. If the client cannot read or has reading deficiencies, the therapist may have to read the book aloud or record it on tape.
5. The client's emotional and chronological age must be considered and reflected in the level of sophistication of the book selected.
6. As Zaccaria and Moses (1968, p. 28) note, reading preferences, both individual and general, are a guideline for book selection:

   Reading preferences of children and adolescents go through a series of predictable stages. From the ages of two or three to about six or seven, children like to have stories read to them concerning familiar events. Then up to the age of ten or eleven years, there is an increasing interest in fantasy stories. Adolescents, too, go through several reading stages. The early adolescent (12-15 years) tends to be interested in animal stories, adventure stories, mystery stories, tales of the supernatural, sports stories. . . . Later on (15-18 years) reading preferences change to such topics as war stories, romance, and stories of adolescent life. Perhaps sparked by the realization that maturity is fast approaching, the reading interests in late adolescence (18-21) tend to focus on such types of stories as those that deal with personal values, social significance, strange and unusual human experiences, and the transition to adult life.

7. Books expressing the same feeling or mood as the client's are often good choices. This principle is called the "isoprinciple" which stems from the technique of music therapy and is commonly used in poetry therapy as well.

8. Audiovisual materials should be considered in treatment if books are not available on a given clinical problem.

CHOOSING BOOKS

Several criteria need to be considered when selecting books for treatment (Coleman and Ganong, 1990). First, the reading level of a book must be matched with the client's reading ability. A book that is too difficult will not be read by the client. A too simple book, in turn, may be insulting to the client.

A second point to be considered is the number of issues and problems covered in the book. Coleman and Ganong (1990) suggest that the more issues dealt with, the better the overall quality of the book. Clients will also more likely read a book that parallels their own experiences.

A third factor is the quality of the advice offered. Ideally, as is the goal of most therapies, a number of possible solutions should be presented. Thus a client, with the support of the practitioner, can use the bibliotherapeutic approach to come up with individualized solutions to the presenting problem.

A fourth area to consider is how realistically the problem is depicted in the book. This point is very important when using fiction as a treatment tool. A well-balanced perspective is very important. Realistic solutions for a problem should be presented in the book.

Finally, the tone of the book should be a consideration. The book or books used in therapy should be nonjudgmental and, if possible, have the valuable quality of humor (Coleman and Ganong, 1990).

Rosen (1981, 1987) adds a number of supporting criteria for choosing books, in particular nonfiction self-help books, for therapeutic intervention. He suggests the therapist should explore the following questions before using a book in treatment.

1. What claims exist in the title of the book that define the it as a do-it-yourself treatment program?
2. Does the book convey accurate information regarding the empirical support for the self-help program?

3. Does the work provide a basis for self-diagnosis, and have the methods for self-diagnosis been evaluated to establish rates of false positives and false negatives?
4. Do the therapeutic techniques in the book have empirical support?
5. Has the book been tested for its clinical efficacy?
6. In light of the above questions, what is the accuracy of any claims made by the author of the book?
7. Can comparisons be made between the book under review and other self-help books on similar topics?

The above questions are intended to help the therapist identify books which have empirical support for the treatment prescribed within the book. In turn, the therapist will have more confidence in the assigned readings to enhance the overall therapeutic process (Pardeck, 1993).

USING BOOKS IN TREATMENT

The following focuses on the use of fiction and self-help books in treatment. Practitioners who prefer fiction are more likely to be grounded in a psychodynamic orientation to therapy; those who have a cognitive-behavioral approach to practice are more apt to use self-help books (Pardeck, 1991b).

Bibliotherapy Through Fiction

Bibliotherapy with clients is often implemented through fiction. When using fiction in treatment, the problem portrayed in a book must be similar to what the client is experiencing. The story and characters are discussed by the therapist and client; this process is designed to find solutions to a presenting problem.

The bibliotherapeutic approach through fiction consists of three phases: *identification and protection, abreaction and catharsis,* and *insight and integration.*

Identification and projection is the first stage of the bibliotherapeutic process. During this stage the therapist helps the client identify with a book character experiencing a problem similar to the client's. The practitioner's role in this process is to assist the client in interpreting the motives of the story character and to provide insight into the relationship among various book characters. During this stage the practitioner helps the client make inferences regarding the meaning of the story and its application to the client's problem (Pardeck, 1991a).

Once identification and projection have occurred, the practitioner moves the client to the *abreaction and catharsis* stage of the bibliotherapeutic process. In order for catharsis to occur, the client must experience an emotional release that is expressed in various ways, including verbal and nonverbal. The involvement of the practitioner at this stage of the treatment process is important and is unique to bibliotherapy versus the normal reading process. During the abreaction and catharsis stage, the therapist must monitor the client's reaction to the reading, the degree of similarity between the client's emotional experience and the problem being treated, and the emotional experiences of the client throughout the process of his or her identification with the book character (Pardeck and Pardeck, 1984).

The final stage of the bibliotherapeutic process is *insight and integration*. During this stage, the client is guided by the therapist to recognize solutions to a problem through the book being read. The client uses this process, with help of the therapits, to develop new strategies for dealing with a confronting problem.

The stages of the bibliotherapy process when using fiction correspond closely to the phases of Freudian psychotherapy. According to Shrodes (1949), a pioneer in the field of bibliotherapy, the process of bibliotherapy involves the following:

> Identification is generally defined as an adaptive mechanism which the human being utilizes, largely unconsciously, to augment his self-regard. It takes the form of a real or imagined affiliation of oneself with another person, a group of persons, or with some institution, or even with a symbol. There is usually involved admiration for the object of one's identification, a tendency to imitate, and a sense of loyalty and belongingness.

> Projection has two common usages in the literature. It consists of the attribution to others of one's own motives or emotions in order to ascribe blame to another instead of to oneself. The term is also used to describe one's perception, apperception, and cognition of the world and people. Catharsis is used synonymously with abreaction to denote the uncensored and spontaneous release of feelings: in the Aristotelian sense it means the purging of emotional awareness of one's motivation, experiences, and subsequent abreaction. (p. 22)

Even though the research findings are mixed on the use of fiction in treatment, many practitioners use this form of bibliotherapy. Fiction has the potential to be a very powerful therapeutic tool because it allows the practitioner and client to do many creative activities in treatment. Suggested activities for working with clients through fiction are covered in Chapter 2.

Self-Help Books

Numerous self-help books have been developed over the last several decades. Therapists will find that self-help books can be an excellent resource for their practice. Self-help books may be used as a technique for offering various options for the client to choose from for dealing with clinical problems. These options will include different strategies for thinking about and coping with a clinical problem. When problem-solving options are offered through books, they can clearly support the therapeutic process. The practitioner may find that if a problem-solving option is offered as a part of the traditional treatment approach, the client may reject it; however, if the therapist has the client read about the option, the client may be more likely to consider it as a serious possibility for solving a problem. This strategy of problem solving is particularly useful for the adolescent client (Coleman and Ganong, 1990).

Self-help books often contain structured activities that clients can do between therapeutic sessions. These activities are designed to encourage problem solving, to stimulate communication between client and therapist, and to help clients identify and process their feelings. These activities can be assigned as homework in therapy, as part of group activities, or as activities during treatment (Coleman and Ganong, 1990).

Self-help books can also be used to stimulate role-playing. Clients can role-play actions described in the books or they can demonstrate ways of responding to situations. After reading a self-help book, clients can brainstorm alternatives from what was read, such as other ways of dealing with the events in the book (Coleman and Ganong, 1990).

There are a number of strategies recommended for using self-help books in treatment (Psychotherapy Newsletter, 1994). These include the following:

- The *self-administered* approach is a treatment strategy that involves the client receiving written material from the practitioner with no additional contact with the therapist beyond the initial session. This approach ends with a final assessment.
- The *minimal-contact* self-help approach involves thc therapist providing reading materials to the client; however, the therapist's role is expanded to written correspondence, phone calls, and infrequent meetings with the client. An example of this approach includes the various weight-control self-help books which involve only minimal contact with the therapist mainly through frequent follow-up calls.
- *Therapist-administered* self-help books are those which the client receives during the beginning of treatment followed by regular meetings with the practitioner. During these meetings, the written materials are discussed and the ways they can be applied to the presenting problem are reviewed.
- The *therapist-directed* approach involves weekly treatment with the therapist. Self-help books are used as part of the weekly treatment. The treatment approach used during the therapeutic session is often reinforced in the self-help book. In some self-help books, self-monitoring forms are available which are designed to help the client to continue to work on a problem between treatment sessions.

Self-help books can be categorized according to the conditions of intended usage. Many self-help books are written in a format that allows individuals to purchase a book over the counter and to implement a plan of intervention without the help of a therapist. This approach obviously is not endorsed by clinicians; however, for certain people confronted with relatively minor adjustment problems, this form of self-help can be useful (Orton, 1997).

The more sound approach to using self-help books in treatment is to involve the therapist at all stages of the treatment process. Many self-help books include self-monitoring forms, descriptions of activities and exercises, and brief summaries of specific procedures that can be used by the therapist as part of treatment. As with all approaches to bibliotherapy, self-help books are designed to be used as an adjunct to treatment (Orton, 1997).

As mentioned previously, those who use fiction in bibliotherapeutic treatment have a tendency to endorse psychodynamic interventions; those practitioners who use self-help books are generally grounded in cognitive-behavioral treatment approaches.

IMPLICATIONS FOR PRACTICE

There are a number of limitations and precautions one should be aware of when using bibliotherapy. One of the most important limitations to bibliotherapeutic intervention is that it should never be used as a single approach to treatment but rather as an adjunct (Pardeck and Pardeck, 1984, 1986; Orton, 1997).

Bibliotherapy as an art has a number of limitations. First, the empirical support for the use of fiction in the bibliotherapeutic approach is mixed; however, the evidence suggests that nonfiction, when used as part of the bibliotherapy process, in the form of self-help books, has sound scientific support. Secondly, individuals who are not inveterate readers may have difficulty benefiting from bibliotherapy. However, bibliotherapy can be conducted successfully with the nonreader through talking books as well as other innovative strategies. Bibliotherapy appears to be most effective with children and adults who are in the habit of reading. Therapists should also know how to judge the client's reading and interest levels. If the match between the client's reading and interest levels is incorrect, the reading material may prove frustrating to the client (Pardeck and Pardeck, 1984).

Another limitation of bibliotherapy is that the client may intellectualize about a problem when reading about it (Giblin, 1989). The client may fail to identify with a character in a fiction book, resulting in a form of projection that can only serve to relieve the client of any responsibility for a resolution to the problem (Pardeck and Pardeck, 1984).

Bernstein (1983) concludes that there is a danger in relying on books too much. Bibliotherapy cannot solve all problems and may even reinforce some problems and promote rationalization in place of change. One must keep in mind that bibliotherapy is not a magical cure for all problems (Pardeck, 1991b; Orton, 1997).

The possibility that the relationship with the therapist and not the reading material is the reason for a client resolving a problem must also be considered (Zaccaria and Moses, 1968). As found for other therapeutic modalities, this can best be monitored by careful assessment of the effect of the therapeutic relationship versus the impact of bibliotherapy on thc client's problem (Pardeck, 1991). If the above points are considered, practitioners will find bibliotherapy to be a creative tool that can support the therapeutic process.

Chapter 2

Clinical Applications of Bibliotherapy

Therapists who wish to use bibliotherapy to help clients deal with problems must consider several factors when selecting books for treatment. The problem the client is facing is the most important issue in book selection. The client's interest and reading levels and alternate forms of book publication must also be considered.

As the definition in Chapter 1 by Barker (1995) suggests, bibliotherapy can be useful for helping clients deal with emotional problems or minor adjustment problems or as a tool for helping clients meet developmental needs. As this book will illustrate later, the practitioner can locate books on many different problem areas facing clients, including emotional problems and developmental needs.

The therapist must consider the client's interest and reading levels as well as the problem facing the client when selecting books for therapy. Age and the level of maturity of the client largely determine the client's interest level. In regard to the client's reading level, a too-difficult book can greatly hamper the bibliotherapeutic process; likewise, a book with a reading level much lower than the client's may prove insulting.

Another consideration of book selection is the form of publication. Numerous books are available in paperback form, which is often more appealing to younger clients. Certain books have been developed in braille and large print; talking books are also available.

The last consideration in book selection is the decision of whether to use fiction or nonfiction in treatment. Fiction includes literature that has been written about a problem. Nonfiction is typically in the form of self-help books. When using fiction in treatment, the client must be able to identify with a book character.

Some nonfiction books may also have book characters. Therefore, fiction or nonfiction books with a biographical character lend themselves most readily to the stages of the bibliotherapeutic process that include *identification and projection, abreaction and catharsis,* and *insight and integration.* These stages of the bibliotherapeutic treatment process are covered in detail in Chapter 1. There are also numerous nonfiction self-help books that offer cognitive-behavioral approaches for dealing with clinical problems.

BIBLIOTHERAPY AND FICTION BOOKS

Figure 2.1 illustrates the procedures for using bibliotherapy through fictional books; however, a number of nonfictional works can also be used with this approach. The bibliotherapy process presented in Figure 2.1 offers a series of distinct activities critical to using books in treatment. These include client readiness and book selection, as well as the client reading the book. Part of the therapeutic process also calls for follow-up activities. These activities are all aimed at moving the client through the stages of the bibliotherapeutic process.

Readiness

Before proceeding with bibliotherapeutic treatment, the therapist must consider an important factor—the client's readiness for biblio-

FIGURE 2.1. Treatment Approach to Bibliotherapy

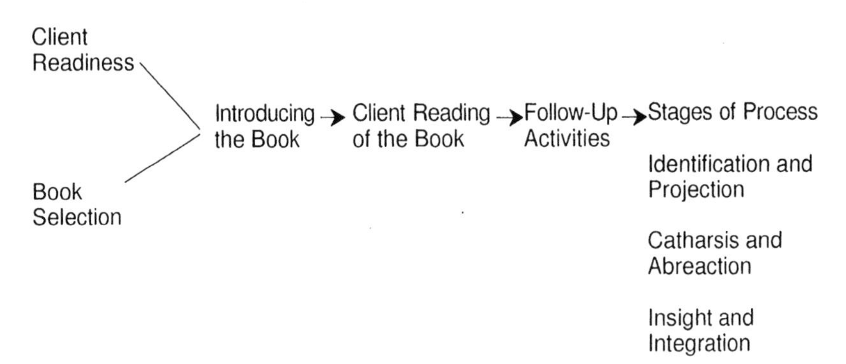

therapy. Inappropriate timing may impede the process. Normally, the client is most ready for the initiation of bibliotherapy when the following conditions have been established: (1) adequate rapport, trust, and confidence have been established between the therapist and the client, (2) the client and therapist have agreed to the presenting problem(s), and (3) some preliminary exploration of the problem has occurred (Orton, 1997).

Selection of Books

The therapist must consider several factors when selecting books for treatment. The most important factor is the presenting problem(s) of the client. The client may be confronted with a minor or major clinical problem. Although books are available on virtually any clinical problem, it is essential that when using fiction that the book contain believable characters and situations that offer realistic hope for the client. The practitioner must also know the client's interest and reading levels. One final element in book selection is the form of publication. Alternative forms such as braille, audiotapes of books, and large type are available for special needs clients. The therapist may wish to use a paperback edition when working with younger clients (Pardeck, 1992).

Introducing the Book

When the client is ready for the bibliotherapeutic process to begin and book selection has been completed, the therapist's next concern is how to introduce the book into treatment. Most practitioners feel that it is best to suggest books rather than to prescribe them; however, one may have to prescribe books for younger clients. Regardless of what strategy the therapist uses for introducing books into therapy, he or she must be familiar with the content of the books selected.

Follow-Up Activities

Orton (1997) emphasizes that effective bibliotherapy includes reading accompanied by discussion and/or counseling. During and after the reading, the client may experience the three stages of the bibliotherapeutic process. Obviously very young clients are not capable of experiencing abreaction and catharsis leading to insight into a clinical problem in the traditional therapeutic sense. For older clients, the advanced stages of the bibliotherapeutic process are important for successful treatment when using fiction and certain kinds of nonfiction books.

The following activities can be utilized by therapists after the book(s) have been read. These follow-up strategies are appropriate for most children and many adults. Certain follow-up activities require a group setting. The practitioner can make use of one activity or several activities. The strategies include creative writing, art activities, discussion, and role-playing (Pardeck and Pardeck, 1987).

Creative Writing

After reading the book, the client might do one or more of the following:

1. Develop a synopsis of the book, using the point of view of a character other than the one who told the story.
2. Make a daily schedule or develop a time line for the character in the story that the client identifies with and compare it to the client's own schedule or time line.
3. Compose a diary for a character in the book.
4. Write a letter from one character in the book to another.
5. Create a different ending to the book or stop reading before the last chapter and come up with an ending.
6. Compose a "Dear Abby" letter that a character in the book could have written about a problem situation.
7. Write a news release focusing on an incident in the book.

Art Activities

Art strategies are better suited for children; however, adults may also benefit from artistic activities. The therapist may wish to follow up the reading of a book by having the client do one or more of the following:

1. Make a map illustrating story events, with the client using his or her imagination to come up with details not given in the book.
2. Construct puppets or make soap or clay models of story characters and reenact a scene from the book.
3. Glue pictures and/or words cut from a magazine on a piece of cardboard to create a collage illustrating the events in the book.
4. Draw pictures in sequence or create a TV scroll of important incidents in the story.
5. Make a mobile that represents key events or characters in the book using the client's own drawings, or pictures cut from a magazine.

Discussion and Role-Playing

The therapist may have the client do one or more of the following:

1. Participate in a group discussion concerning a decision that presents itself to one of the book characters.
2. Role-play an incident in the book, with the client taking the part of a key character.
3. Hold a mock trial concerning an incident in the story, with the clients playing the parts of defendant, lawyers, judge, jury, and witnesses.
4. Discuss the strong and weak points of a character with whom the client identifies.

The therapist can adapt the activities to fit each client; for example, a client who dislikes writing can use a tape recorder for the creative writing activities. Depending on the client's problem and the type of book used, the therapist may wish to suggest several follow-up activities from which the client can select one or more.

BIBLIOTHERAPY AND SELF-HELP BOOKS

As presented in Chapter 1, self-help books can be used by therapists through the following approaches: *self-administered, minimal-*

contact, therapist-administered, and *therapist-directed.* Each of these strategies call for different levels of involvement by a therapist in the treatment process.

Even though no specific model has emerged for using self-help books in treatment, Craighead, McNamara, and Horan (1984) offer a general model that clinicians might find useful:

1. Specific techniques offered in the book are the primary ingredient of the therapeutic relationship.
2. Techniques in the book must be in language the client can read and understand.
3. Techniques must be standardized; that is, they are applicable to many individuals, not only one.
4. The suggested techniques must have a relatively low risk level.
5. The individual is considered capable of selecting a self-help book and has the right to be involved in the selection of the goals of treatment.
6. Individuals are considered to be capable of self-instructed change; however, the therapist can greatly facilitate the self-help process.

What this basic model suggests is that individuals should be empowered to make decisions about their own lives. Furthermore, one might argue that the model is grounded in two scientific theories, specifically, behavioral and cognitive theories of intervention (Pardeck, 1993).

Skinner (1953) concluded that individuals have the ability to control their own behavior. In the behavioral therapeutic tradition, individual behavior is largely determined by external factors. Homme's (1965) cognitive view suggests that "operants of the mind" trigger attempts to extend self-control procedures to include changes in thoughts as well as individual behavior. Many self-help books are grounded in the behavioral and cognitive theoretical traditions. Most self-help books stress changing or modifying one's environment if the problem is triggered by environmental forces. Self-help books often offer self-monitoring exercises, self-evaluation, and self-reinforcements. These are therapeutic techniques stressed in behavioral and cognitive treatment approaches (Pardeck, 1993).

Ellis (1993) even argues that self-help books may be more effective for clients than treatment from a clinical practitioner. Ellis suggests that self-help books can be viewed as a medium that empowers people because the control of therapy shifts from the practitioner to the client. It must be noted, however, that this is a view not widely held by professionals in the field of mental health.

SELF-HELP BOOKS IN TREATMENT

Self-help books are typically nonfictional works that offer strategies for cognitive, emotional, and behavioral change. A number of strategies can be used to help ensure the effectiveness of self-help books. The use of these various strategies is greatly determined by how a self-help book is utilized in treatment.

Timing

When to include a self-help book in the treatment process must be carefully planned by the practitioner. The practitioner should carefully prepare and plan before offering a self-help book to a client. It is critical for the client to have choices in determining what books will be used. A self-help book should never be forced upon the client, as if it were medicine, but rather offered as a resource that empowers the client. The client must be ready and willing to use books in treatment to ensure that this form of bibliotherapy is successful (Pardeck, 1993).

For example, when grieving is at its peak, it is difficult for individuals to effectively deal with this emotion. Even though the presenting problem is known to the client and therapist, emotional relief is first needed in other areas of social functioning. However, until the client is ready, it is very difficult to confront the grief directly. If a therapist is not sensitive to the issue of timing and a book is introduced at an inappropriate time, the client's fears, guilt, and depression may be intensified through the self-help book (Pardeck, 1993).

Discussion

A self-help book must first be read before it is discussed. It should be noted that a great deal can be learned by simply reading the self-help book without discussing it with anyone. Simply reading a self-help book can lead to self growth and development.

Still, one of the most important aspects of using self-help books in therapy is discussing the book with the therapist. It is critical for the therapist to listen with empathy. This allows the client maximum opportunity to express feelings and various emotions about a problem. This process also creates trust between the therapist and client. Trust, respect, and empathy are all critical components of successful therapy (Rogers, 1969).

Preparation

Prior to using a self-help book in therapy, Bernstein (1989) suggests a number of factors that need to be considered. The first is the practitioner should read the book. Other critical steps include exploring the following questions:

- What is the scope of the self-help book?
- Is the book accurate, or is there information that must be clarified?
- Will the book have an emotional impact on the client?
- What is the religious or moral tone of the book?
- Is the self-help book worthwhile from a literary viewpoint; that is, will it satisfy the reader on an emotional and verbal level, and possibly even a spiritual level?
- Is the self-help book appropriate for the individual's age, interests, and reading level?
- Will the self-help book's length, format, or level of difficulty prevent clinical gains?
- Is the self-help book in keeping with the reader's general developmental life tasks, such as someone entering marriage or having a first child?
- Does the client have special needs; that is, does he or she need large print or an audio book, or does the client have a limited vocabulary, which means sensitivity to the reading level of the book?

CRITICAL ISSUES

The popularization of self-help books and the prediction of an increased role of books in treatment are important issues that should be explored before introducing books in treatment. These specifically deal with the negative effects of self-help approaches.

Santrock, Minnett, and Campbell (1994) found that some self-help books tend to attack mental health professionals. Others offer utopian or single solutions to problems that are simply unrealistic. Practitioners must be careful not to recommend these kinds of books to clients because they can contribute to dissatisfaction and even make presenting problems worse.

Practitioners should also be sensitive to ineffective programs offered in self-help books. This is obviously an important concern for individuals who are deciding on a self-administered program. Even though consumers have a right to choose, they may lack the necessary information to choose wisely. Ineffective programs may erode consumer confidence in self-help books and may ultimately impact the trust levels of professional practitioners. Ineffective self-help books may actually exacerbate clinical problems. It is critical for therapists and consumers to study the claims made by a self-help book program. If a consumer cannot make an appropriate judgment about the quality of a self-help book, he or she should ask a professional about the effectiveness of a given self-help program (Pardeck, 1993).

Finally, for those who use self-administered programs, inappropriate self-diagnosis is always a potential problem. When using a self-administered program, the reader must determine both the type and severity of a presenting problem. An inaccurate self-diagnosis may result in a person choosing a self-administered program, when a more intensive therapeutic approach is needed. A reasonable solution to this potential problem is for the practitioner to provide the needed assistance to clients at all stages of a self-help program. Consumers of self-help books must carefully choose an appropriate self-help program and seek professional guidance if they are not sure about a particular self-administered program (Pardeck, 1993).

Quackenbush (1991) concludes that therapists must be aware of a number of ethical issues related to self-help books, including authors lacking professional credentials who write self-help materials. Such issues need to be carefully considered by professionals and consumers. Finally, self-help books appear to be within the ethical standards of most helping professions as long as they have an education-training context or personal advice from a professional who is a licensed therapist.

BIBLIOTHERAPY AND GROUP TREATMENT

Bibliotherapy can be used as part of group treatment. The practitioner can use both fictional and nonfiction books in group settings. Therapists can use the bibliotherapy approach as an intervention activity in the following kinds of groups: recreational, educational, therapeutic, and personal growth groups (Pardeck, 1996).

The goal of the recreational group is pure enjoyment. This kind of group often does not have a leader and activities are typically spontaneous. Examples of recreational group activities include playground activities, game room activities, and informal baseball, volleyball, or football groups. The recreational group is often viewed as a system that prevents juvenile delinquency and builds character. Recreational reading can be done in this kind of setting.

The educational group is a small group system that helps participants acquire knowledge and learn complex skills. Leaders of this form of group are well trained and are often professionals. Educational groups focus on a variety of topics including training foster parents, teaching parenting techniques, and training volunteers for specialized functions with human service systems. Social workers are often leaders of educational groups and can include reading materials as part of the educational process. When working with educational groups, therapists are encouraged to involve group members in discussion and in-depth group interaction.

The therapeutic group is an advanced form of group work that attempts to deal with unconscious motivation and behavioral change of group members. Group therapy is often of long-term duration and include clients with severe emotional disabilities. Group therapy is conducted in schools, institutions, and mental health centers. Practitioners leading group therapy are highly trained professionals grounded in advanced knowledge and skills of small group interaction. There are countless books available for conducting bibliotherapy in the therapeutic group setting.

The personal growth group is often composed of healthy people who wish to improve their lives. They seek to improve communication skills, develop leadership skills, improve relationship skills, and develop personal attitudes or abilities of group members. They attempt to encourage growth by helping group members to reassess their potential and to act positively on this reassessment. Classic examples of personal growth groups include the encounter and integrity groups. Many self-help books are designed specifically for use in the personal growth group.

Groups are a powerful tool for changing emotions and behaviors in clients (Wang and Walberg, 1985). Groups that are designed to change a client's social functioning can not only teach new coping strategies but also offer support.

Groups can serve many purposes in professional settings. As therapists realize, groups can be a powerful tool for helping to heal emotional problems and change problem behaviors. In essence, when using bibliotherapy in a group setting, the total being of a client can be affected.

A number of issues must be considered when using bibliotherapy in a group setting. These issues mainly apply to groups that are designed to help clients improve their social functioning.

Communication

By participating in a group setting, clients can improve their communication skills. This process may also help contribute to the client's total well-being and, in particular, increase the client's self-esteem.

Learning

As clients share their feelings in a group setting, they not only improve their communication and relationship skills, but also learn new coping behaviors. Clients learn to deal more effectively with their own feelings and also how to contribute to the group process.

Insight

A group setting can increase the client's awareness of self, enhance self-understanding, and provide him or her with solutions to problems.

Expression

The group setting may be viewed as a specialized laboratory where feelings that normally might be taboo in a conventional context are allowed and ventilated, thus providing a client with a meaningful release or catharsis.

Orientation

A group approach to intervention can be viewed as an orienting device, facilitating each group member's readiness to learn new materials. The group helps clients to stay focused and to accomplish group goals.

BOOKS, HUMAN DEVELOPMENT, AND GROUPS

As noted in Chapter 1, bibliotherapy has been known by a number of different names including bibliocounseling, biblioeducation, bibliopsychology, and literatherapy. Thompson and Rudolph (1996) conclude that bibliotherapy is a family of techniques for structuring interaction between a clinician and a participant based on mutual sharing of reading material.

Orton (1997) suggests that bibliotherapy can be used as a powerful tool by therapists to enhance behavioral growth and development of individuals. When books are used in treatment, trust between the client and therapist grows. Once this mutual trust is established, the client finds it easier to cope with threatening moments and tension during the treatment process. The trusting bond between client and therapist is critical to the bibliotherapeutic process. The creative use of books in treatment can enhance such a bond.

Bibliotherapy can also be viewed as a useful tool for helping clients cognitively restructure a clinical problem. It is assumed that once clients have enough information about a problem, certain positive outcomes will occur. Outcomes that can positively impact a client's social functioning include the following:

1. The client can become psychologically and emotionally involved with characters read about.
2. A client can be taught constructive and positive thinking.
3. Reading can encourage free expression concerning the problem.
4. The client can be helped to analyze attitudes and behaviors through reading.
5. Reading can help a client find solutions to a problem.
6. Through reading, the client can see similarities between his or her own problem and those of others.
7. Books can help a person accept a problem and offer new and creative ways for dealing with it.

Bibliotherapy can facilitate the group process because the goals of bibliotherapy support the traditional approaches to group treatment. In particular, Pardeck and Pardeck (1987) conclude that bibliotherapy teaches clients the following:

1. It enhances positive thinking for individuals. For the disconnected person, positive thinking can lead to improved self-esteem.
2. It encourages free expression, a goal critical to individual and group intervention. Obviously this process enhances the growth and development of all group members.
3. Through the bibliotherapeutic process clients learn to analyze their attitudes and behaviors. This process is clearly critical to the group process.
4. When using bibliotherapy in a group setting, clients may find solutions to personal problems and develop strategies for dealing effectively with them in the future.

Consequently, the goals of bibliotherapy can support a group approach to treatment. The creative use of bibliotherapy in a group setting can enhance the social and emotional development of clients (Pardeck and Pardeck, 1989).

GROUP SKILLS AND BIBLIOTHERAPY

A number of interpersonal skills are critical to the group process (Johnson and Johnson, 1975, 1981). Skills the practitioner emphasizes depend on the needs of the clients. The following list of skills offers a practitioner a starting point for examining where clients are in terms of functioning in the group setting. The four skill levels are as follows:

1. *Forming:* The most basic skill needed for functioning in a group setting.
2. *Functioning:* The skills needed to manage the group process in completing the task and maintaining an effective working relationship among group members.
3. *Formulating:* The skills needed to build a deeper level of understanding among group members, to stimulate the use of higher quality reasoning strategies, and to master and retain information acquired during the group process.
4. *Fermenting:* The skills needed to stimulate reconceptualization of the group experience, including the cognitive and emotional conflict members experienced during the group process.

Forming Skills

The basic skills, or forming skills, should be taught to help clients to organize the group and establish minimum standards of appropriate group behavior. Clients must be encouraged to respect others in the group and to help all participants involved in the group process. Other necessary basic group skills that should be encouraged are to address group members by their first names; to be positive toward other group members; and finally, to keep focused on group goals.

Functioning Skills

These important skills include managing the group's efforts to complete tasks and to be an effective working group. Clients have to learn to stay with the tasks and to set time limits. They must also learn to show support for each other verbally and nonverbally as well as know how to ask for help and clarification for what is being said or done in the group. Clients must also learn to express their feelings and to motivate other group members.

Formulating Skills

This set of skills is needed to provide the mental processes needed to build deeper understanding of the books being read, to stimulate the use of higher quality reasoning, and to ensure mastery of the assigned materials in books. Particularly, the clients master how to summarize aloud what has been read. The clients learn to ask other group members to relate materials covered to other things with which they are familiar. They learn to seek ways to remember the important ideas and facts presented in various books read. Finally, the clients master how to vocalize the implicit reasoning process used by the group to complete assigned tasks.

Fermenting Skills

Fermenting refers to the skills needed to stimulate reconceptualization of the books being used in intervention, cognitive conflict, and the communication of the rationale behind the group's behavior. Important learning tasks take place when the clients master how to challenge each other's conclusions and reasoning. This process moves the group deeper into the book, to think more divergently about issues offered in the book, and to move toward solutions that can help clients with confronting problems.

Skills specifically mastered through the process of fermenting include: clients learn how to criticize issues, not people; they learn how to integrate a number of different ideas into a single position; clients learn how to ask group members to justify a conclusion as well as to extend another group member's answer or conclusion by adding further information or implications; finally, clients learn how to probe other group members through asking questions that result in a deeper understanding and analysis of a problem.

CONSIDERATIONS OF CONDUCTING BIBLIOTHERAPY WITH GROUPS

A number of steps should be considered before implementing bibliotherapy in a group setting. The first step is the selection of the books to be read by group members, with attention given to interest and reading levels. The composition of a group, group rules, task setting, and follow-up activities must all be considered. The therapist may also wish to prepare a means for evaluating the group process.

Selecting Books

When using bibliotherapy with groups, the books selected should deal with a general theme that all group members can identify with, such as making new acquaintances, getting along with others, or improving one's self-esteem (Pardeck and Pardeck, 1989). Practitioners who have a range of choices when forming groups might select books dealing with more specific problems, such as grouping together clients who are experiencing divorce. Hardbound or paperback books are often available in sets according to a theme or certain author. Keep in mind that the practitioner needs a book for each group member, so it may be necessary to make sure multiple copies of a book title are available.

There must also be consideration of the individual needs and characteristics of group members. Group members need to be fairly close in age chronologically or at approximately the same developmental level so that any books selected will be suitable for all group members. The reading level of each individual must be known so that any book selected will not be too difficult for the lowest level reader in the group. High-interest low-vocabulary books are a good choice for those with reading problems. Many books are available on cassette tapes, or the clinician might record a book as an option for the client with obvious reading difficulties.

Suggestions for Starting and Maintaining Groups

Much of the first session will be needed to establish group rules and explain the purpose of the group. This is when clients become familiar with forming skills. Rules should be kept simple and should be covered in the first group session. Group rules should stress cooperation and participation by all group members. If more than one group will be working at one time, it must be stressed that groups must not disturb each another. The size of each group should range from three to five members.

At the beginning of all group sessions, the clinician should make a statement of what the group should accomplish. This can be posted and called "Tasks for Today." This way, clients are well aware of the goals of a given session. The clinician may want to set time limits for tasks during the first few sessions, in particular. For example, the therapist might tell group members who have spent five minutes retelling a chapter to move to the next task required. Eventually groups who have progressed to functioning skills should be able to set their own time limits.

For groups needing leadership, the group member who is thought by the practitioner to have the strongest leadership skills should be selected to be the writer (leader) during the first session. This person tries to keep the group on task and reads aloud any written directions for group tasks. The writer (leader) also writes down answers to questions for the whole group, making sure he or she obtains at least one response from each group member. Everyone in the group should eventually have a chance to be the group leader.

Follow-Up Activities

As mentioned previously, there is agreement among virtually all studies on bibliotherapy that the reading of a book must be accompanied by discussion or other activities. When posting tasks to be completed during a group session, the therapist may wish to begin with either oral or silent reading and then provide a transition with a follow-up activity. Examples of writing and thinking activities, particularly when using fiction in treatment, that can be employed by the clinician as a follow-up to a book or book chapter include the following:

1. Making predictions before the reading of a book. These predictions might be based on the book title, cover illustrations, or chapter titles.

2. Answering questions about details after each chapter. Strategies for locating answers to Who, What, When, and Where questions could be reviewed by the group.
3. Role-playing the actions and conversations of characters in a chapter. When using fiction in treatment, this might lead to a better comprehension by the clients of character emotions and motives.
4. Using context clues to complete a paragraph with vocabulary from a chapter. Depending on the skill level of the group, the therapist may want to provide the first letter of the missing word or have a list of vocabulary words to choose from.
5. Checking on earlier predictions after reading the first few chapters of the book. The therapist can decide which predictions have proved to be correct.
6. Creating a time line of story events after reading a few chapters or after completing the entire book. This might increase a client's understanding of sequencing or putting events in order.
7. Determining cause-effect relationships within a chapter or several chapters. This can either be a matching exercise or a diagram with fill-in boxes for clients to complete.
8. Thinking up a different ending for a book. Clients can collaborate on other ways the story might have ended.
9. Comparing two major characters after reading a book. Similarities and differences between the characters can be listed by the clients.
10. Composing a letter or telegram to one of the book's characters. Clients can work on this with the skill of summarizing the entire book in mind.

After a number of sessions, groups can ultimately move toward formulating and fermenting skills through the use of follow-up activities such as those listed above. It should also be noted that a number of self-help books are available that are specifically designed for group settings (Doll and Doll, 1997). Many of the group activities offered above can also be used with self-help books.

In conclusion, the use of bibliotherapy in a group setting is useful for clients of all ages and intellectual levels. As with any therapeutic technique, however, the practitioner must use good judgment in the application of bibliotherapy in the group setting. Few therapists would deny that reading problem-centered books has considerable value in helping clients deal with growth and developmental needs. It is more than evident that unique needs of clients call for new innovations in treatment such as bibliotherapy in a group setting. Such therapeutic innovations not only enhance the intellectual development of clients, but also their emotional and social development.

CONCLUSION

Fiction and nonfiction books are widely used by clinical practitioners. Practitioners grounded in psychodynamic approaches to treatment have a tendency to use fiction in treatment; those who employ behavioral-cognitive treatment techniques tend to use nonfiction self-help books in therapy. Strategies for using fiction and nonfiction are presented in this chapter as well as a detailed discussion for using bibliotherapy in a group setting.

A great deal of research has been conducted on bibliotherapy, and self-help books grounded in behavioral-cognitive theories are considered to have the greatest efficacy as treatment tools. Given these findings, therapists should be aware of the strengths and limitations of books in treatment. Even though additional research needs to be conducted on the effectiveness of bibliotherapy, Starker (1988) reports that books are widely used in treatment by mental health professionals. Riordan (1991, p. 306) succinctly summarizes the current state of using books in treatment:

> Many of us find colleagues of differing orientations using articles, book chapters, poems, or other references to clarify, instruct, reinforce, or otherwise assist in therapy. The pertinent issue is not really whether bibliotherapy is effective as a separate therapy, but rather what, when, and how it should be use as part of a treatment plan.

Chapter 3

Clinical Problems and Bibliotherapy

This chapter offers a brief overview of a number of problem areas that often confront individuals and their families. These areas include divorce and remarriage, dysfunctional families, parenting, self-development, serious illness, and substance-related disorders. Chapter 4 offers annotated summaries of books that can be used as tools to help clients deal with each of these problem areas. Sample books and a case study are presented in this chapter on the problem of divorce. The quality of books available for the problem area of divorce is representative of the books found in other clinical areas. The case study illustrates how bibliotherapy can be used with a child dealing with the divorce of his parents.

DIVORCE AND REMARRIAGE

Research suggests the family experiencing divorce needs additional support (Pardeck, 1990). Increasing numbers of children and adults are experiencing family breakdown because of divorce (Gardner, 1984). A key concern for many parents who divorce is the impact that it has on their children. Orton (1997) reports that children of divorce are often confronted with a number of unique problems that should be recognized and resolved. In particular, children often have problems acknowledging the divorce, resolving the loss related to it, dealing with anger and self-blame, accepting the permanence of the divorce, and finally, forming relationships with others. Research by Wallerstein and Blakeslee (1989) suggests that many of these feelings are long term. For example, adults who experienced divorce as children often have unresolved anger because of family breakdown, have a history of underachievement in school, and have problems forming close relationships. These findings suggest that divorce is a difficult process for children to deal with and that problems related to divorce should be resolved as early as possible in the child's life (Orton, 1997).

Parents must realize that a child's adjustment to divorce often takes time and requires effort by all significant adults in the child's life. Thompson and Rudolph (1996) suggest that group counseling is helpful for not only children of divorce but also their parents. As illustrated in Chapter 2, books can be a helpful adjunct to the group intervention process.

Even as the family system changes within the United States (Pardeck, 1993), practitioners must remember that the intact nuclear family traditionally has been viewed as the *ideal* family system. As divorce and remarriage rates increase, the structure and nature of the modern family must be reconsidered. Thompson and Rudolph (1996) conclude that approximately one-third of all children born in the 1990s will live in blended families. The blended family system is a family in which at least one adult has had a child prior to the couple's marriage (Orton, 1997).

The joining of two families into one creates problems and new challenges for children and their parents. For example, children in blended families often must cope with the effects of their biological parents' divorce. For parents, the stigma of failure in their first marriage may also be problematic. Given these conditions, members of blended families bring a unique set of problems and concerns to the therapeutic setting. Practitioners who work with blended families must work with adults and children who are often still dealing with problems related to a prior marriage. Furthermore, clinicians must work with problems in blended families that are very different from problems of first marriage families (Pardeck, 1993).

Research suggests that blended families are not necessarily problematic; rather they are different from biological families in ways that need to be accepted and recognized (Kelly, 1992). Duncan and Brown (1992), in fact, point out the many strengths found in blended families which include: positive communication, caring, pride, unity, and ties with their extended families and communities. Even though there are numerous strengths found in blended families, family members may bring emotional baggage from their families of origin, from first marriages, and from the process of divorce and remarriage (Whitsett and Land, 1992a, 1992b).

Orton (1997) has identified a number of issues that practitioners need to consider when working with blended families. First, children in blended families often fear they will lose their biological parent's time and affection. It is not uncommon for children to worry that their parent will be less available when he or she remarries. Second, stepparents are never a substitute for biological parents. Stepparents must be aware of the strong emotional attachments that children will continue to have for the absent parent. Third, loyalty conflicts are greater for older children. Wallerstein and Blakeslee (1989) found that 50 percent of older children resented their stepfathers; the majority had difficulty accepting stepfathers as authority figures. Fourth, positive relationships do not happen overnight; the development of healthy parent-child relationships takes time. Last, stepparent relationships can be successful. When trust develops between stepparent and children, genuine love and affection can result.

Orton (1997, pp. 112-113) suggests the following strategies for working with parents of divorce and blended families:

1. Encourage parents to talk to their children about divorce and how it will affect their lives.
2. Reassure children that they did not cause the divorce.
3. Recognize and treat children's grief related to the loss of their intact family.
4. Recognize that children can adapt to their new families; however, this will take time.
5. Include biological parents and stepparents in counseling.
6. Help parents support their children through the difficult time of forming a new family.

If practitioners keep the above issues in mind when working with children and their parents, transition to a blended family can evolve more smoothly.

There are many myths about blended families of which practitioners must be aware. Also, blended families have strengths and weaknesses like all family systems. Still, the practitioner should be aware of the unique problems that face the blended family versus other family systems.

The self-help books offered in Chapter 4 are designed to help parents and children deal with the unique problems associated with divorce and the creation of the blended family. The sources listed and annotated in Chapter 4 can be used in individual counseling, group settings, or simply as a resource for families to better understand problems associated with divorce and remarriage.

DYSFUNCTIONAL FAMILIES

A great deal of theory has emerged that is critical of explaining problems related to individual social functioning through an individual pathology approach (Hepworth, Rooney, and Larsen, 1997). Recent theories for understanding and explaining problems related to individual social functioning are heavily grounded in the ecological perspective (DuBois and Miley, 1996). To fully understand problems related to social functioning, one must look at the individual, familial, social, and cultural factors that all play a part in the creation of problems that confront people in their daily lives (Pardeck, 1996).

Research suggests that family dysfunction plays a major role in contributing to problems related to individual social functioning. Hartman (1994) suggests that pressures inside and outside the family system help define the emotional well-being of family members. Families that have the ability to adapt and change will greatly determine how stress is managed by the family system. Families that do not adapt to pressures are likely to experience dysfunctions including child abuse, violence, and substance abuse (Hartman, 1994).

Child abuse is a serious problem often associated with the dysfunctional family. The National Research Council (1993) identified the following signs often associated with child abuse: injuries that cannot be explained as accidental; lack of trust; fearful, shy, and withdrawn behavior; aggressive behavior; acting-out behavior; extreme difficulty in verbalizing feelings; feelings of profound sadness; poor self-esteem; excessive fears, sleep disturbances, and regressive behavior; and an incapacity to play at acceptable developmental levels with other children.

The following are guidelines for working with abused children. First, the practitioner should help the abused child, through the treatment process, to begin to trust others. Second, the practitioner needs to be a positive role model by demonstrating consistent and positive behavior when interacting with the child. Third, attention must be given to building and enhancing the child's self-esteem. The child must be taught to feel good about him or herself before effective therapy can proceed. Finally, the child must be encouraged to talk about the abuse experience. Bibliotherapy can be a particularly effective tool for assisting children in expressing their feelings about the abuse (Orton, 1997).

Domestic violence is another problem associated with dysfunctional families. *Battering* is a form of physical violence perpetrated by one person on another and typically includes a life-threatening history of injury and psychosocial problems that trap a person in a relationship. Battering is not confined to heterosexual relationships; gays and lesbians are not immune to battering one another (Coleman, 1994; Dutton, 1994). Furthermore, physical abuse of women is not confined only to the husband-wife relationship; single, separated, or divorced women are at greater risk than married women for battering (Marino, 1994).

Abusive men tend to have certain traits (Walker, 1989). They often have poor communication skills, unrealistic expectations for their spouse or partner, and lack self-control. It is common for them to be dependent on and possessive toward their spouse or partner. Often they have problems with alcohol and drugs. Many were abused as children. Last, abusive men often feel a lack of comparative power to women in economic status, decision making, and communication skills.

Women in battering relationships appear to have common characteristics as well (Walker, 1989). They tend to have low self-esteem and feelings of inadequacy. They have a history of abuse that leads them to accept their role as victim. The physical and emotional wounds of battering often cause these victims to become physically and emotionally isolated. They sometimes have problems asserting their rights and feelings. Finally, battered women often lack personal, physical, educational, and financial resources that would allow them to leave the battering situation.

Books are included in Chapter 4 that deal with problems found in dysfunctional families. Many of the books focus on the emotional and behavioral problems associated with child abuse. Other books deal with problems related to families under pressure, including family violence.

PARENTING

The pressures of working, finding appropriate day care, and meeting the needs of children are some of the more difficult tasks confronting parents on a daily basis. There are a number of clearly predictable crises that come with parenthood. One crisis is the birth of the first child. Many life transitions must be made by new parents. One transition is that adulthood becomes "official"; new parents must care not only for themselves, but also a new baby. The arrival of a newborn means tweny-four-hour care since a baby demands a tremendous amount of attention. If parents work, their schedules must change, while new roles and responsibilities emerge that have never been dealt with before. Even in the most enlightened families, the bulk of caring for children falls on the mother. Although increasing numbers of men—particularly those in dual-career families with young children—are helping with child care and housework (Papalia and Olds, 1996), women are still responsible for the lion's share (Schor, 1992).

Even though children bring great joy to parents, they are also an economic liability. Thus, parenting has both a negative and positive impact on one's lifestyle. Given the fact that children are an economic liability, modern families have a tendency to be small. Even though attitudes toward marriage and parenting have changed over the years, many couples still feel compelled by the larger society to have children (Pardeck, 1993).

Parents have a profound effect on a child's personality development. Children are influenced by the style of coping with life that the parent models, the quality of the parents' interaction with the child, and how parents treat a child based on the child's place in the family system. Furthermore, a child's behavior is affected by interaction of the family system as a whole. If the family environment is healthy, the child has a greater chance of positive growth and development. If the family environment is unhealthy, children often suffer.

Thompson and Rudolph (1996) stress that parenting styles have a major impact on a child's emotional and social development. Families often exhibit one of three basic types of parenting: authoritarian, authoritative, and laissez-faire. Children who experience the same type of parenting style often have common characteristics.

The *authoritarian* parenting style is restrictive and punitive. Parents who use this style permit little give and take with children and place many limits on the children's behavior. This kind of parenting is linked with children who show high levels of anxiety, ineffective social interaction with others, and social underdevelopment in a number of areas.

Authoritative parenting is an approach that encourages independence; however, it places limits and demands on the child's behavior. There is much verbal give and take, and parents demonstrate a high degree of warmth and support toward their children. Children who experience this type of parenting style often will exhibit greater social competency, self-reliance, and social responsibility.

When parents use a *laissez-faire* approach to child rearing, they place low demands, limits, and controls on their children's behavior. This parenting style provides children considerable freedom, while parents take a nonpunitive stance. Parents using a laissez-faire style are not very involved with their children. Children raised with this kind of parenting tend to be immature, regressive, and unable to assume leadership positions.

Developmental specialists continue to stress the influence that parenting style has on children's emotional and social development (Orton, 1997). Considering the styles presented here, the authoritative style includes an approach that sets limits yet delivers warmth and respect. This appears to be far superior to the other approaches.

The parenting process has four distinct stages (Pardeck, 1993). These include *anticipation, the honeymoon, the plateau,* and *disengagement.*

Anticipation occurs during pregnancy and involves the parents beginning to think about how they will raise their child. Expectant parents are often nervous about their new role and are uncertain about what it will involve. Expectant parents are often uncertain about how effective they will be in the parenting role.

The honeymoon stage occurs after the child is born. It normally lasts for several months. During the honeymoon stage, parents are usually happy to have a new baby and enjoy providing for the child. This stage is a time of adjustment and learning; bonding begins between parents and child, and new roles are learned by parents.

The plateau stage begins at infancy and lasts through adolescence. It is a time of adjustment for both parents and their children. The skills needed for parenting are different at each phase of the child's development during this stage.

Disengagement occurs when children leave home. When a child leaves home for marriage or for other reasons, such as college, the parent-child relationship goes through a dramatic change, evolving to an adult-adult relationship.

These stages suggest children have a great effect on parents. In turn, parents obviously have a tremendous influence on a child's social development. It must be recognized, however, that other systems influence a child's development, including the peer group. Consequently, a child's development is not totally determined by interaction with parents through the family life cycle.

Adoption

Adoption calls for an awareness of the unique problems that adoptive children frequently must face. Special parenting skill are critical to help children deal with the problems related to the adoption process. Adoptive parents must help the child realize that he or she will not be returning to his or her biological family. Even if the child has been in an extended foster care placement, the child may continue to fantasize about returning to the biological family. Adoptive parents must help the child work through this fantasy, which will not be given up easily. Gradually, the fantasy will be abandoned. This may result in the child entering a stage of mourning for his or her biological parents. If this stage occurs, the child will need help to express anger and pain when reminiscing about his or her past, and must be helped to realize that he or she will not return to the biological family. Open and truthful discussion of the child's past is the most effective approach; denial and secrecy may be emotionally damaging to the child (Pardeck, 1990).

Melina (1989, pp. 5-7) stresses that practitioners need to be sensitive to the basic rights to which all adoptive children should be entitled. These include the following:

- Having a right to know who they are and how they joined their families, and to grow up knowing the truth about their adoption
- Having a right to freely ask questions and express their feelings about being adopted
- Having a right to a positive attitude about the birth parents
- Having a right to be recognized by society as full and equal members of their adoptive families
- Having a right to information about their origins
- Having a right to a positive sense of racial or ethnic identity (if transracially adopted)

The research literature strongly suggests that allowing adoptive children these basic rights will enhance their growth and development (Hepworth, Rooney, and Larsen, 1997).

Once the child is placed in an adoptive home, fantasies of returning to the biological family may continue and the need to connect to the past continues to be an important psychological factor. Adoptive parents should realize that adopted children, especially those who have been abused or who are older, may be fearful, angry, and anticipating another rejection. Initial placement in an adoptive setting will often go smoothly; this period of tranquillity, however, may be artificial because the child has not yet bonded with the adopted family. This "honeymoon" period often ends when the adoptive child begins to feel stirrings of caring and longing which bring back old emotions. The child may resist bonding with the adoptive family because he or she is frightened of another rejection by significant others. This difficult time can be reframed, however, as an indication that the child is beginning to care about the adoptive parents. Such a transition is difficult for both the child and the adoptive parents (Orton, 1997).

Children who experience adoption have many special needs. A move to a new home involves separation from the family with whom they have lived; they must establish a relationship within an unknown new family; and, for most children, old separation issues are reworked, particularly those involving the child's biological family. Children undergoing separation from their birth and foster families commonly experience denial, anger, and depression. They may feel sadness because they are losing their biological or foster families, and at the same time experience fear and anxiety about the future. It is not unusual for the adoptive child to also feel anger because he or she is placed in a situation that causes confusing emotions (Rudman, Gagne, and Berstein, 1993).

Foster Care

Some children must be placed in foster care. DuBois and Miley (1996, p. 407) note that the typical reasons for placement include the following:

1. Parents are unable to continue their caretaker responsibilities.
2. Parents have neglected or abused their children.
3. Parents are absent due to death, abandonment, or incarceration.
4. Parents have a serious physical or emotional disability.
5. The children have behavioral, personality, or physical problems that necessitate placement.

Regardless of the reasons for placement, children in foster care often experience confusion and trauma when separated from their families. After children are placed in care, the child welfare system aims its services at reunification.

Children placed in foster care typically will live with a foster family. However, for certain children, the placement of choice may be in an institutional setting, a residential setting, or a group home. These kinds of living arrangements are often used for older or special-needs children (Hepworth, Rooney, and Larsen, 1997).

One of the major problems that foster children encounter is the separation from their biological parents. Foster children must know that their biological parents will visit them regularly and that the goal is to return them to their families. However, for some children a return home is not possible, and it is critical for the child to have a sense of permanency in the most family-like environment possible (Hepworth, Rooney, and Larsen, 1997).

Foster care also involves new roles, positions, and realignments within foster families. These changes within the foster family must be recognized and dealt with by the foster parents. Children who have been placed in foster care because of abuse or neglect may be especially troubled children. It is important for all foster children to be able to express their feelings related to their placement, and to be provided with the opportunity to resolve the conflicts related to these feelings. The practitioner, as well as foster parents or other caretakers, is a critical part of this process (Rudman, Gagne, and Berstein, 1993).

The books annotated in Chapter 4 on parenting are aimed not only at parents raising biological children but also at those who care for adopted and foster children. The children in these special families have needs similar to those found in other families; however, there are also unique differences. The titles offered provide parents and practitioners with helpful strategies for parenting and raising children in various kinds of settings.

SELF-DEVELOPMENT

Self-development is a lifelong process. Self-development involves improving communication skills, improving assertion and personal relationship skills, improving leadership skills, and improving positive thinking about oneself and others. Even though self-development is largely aimed at emotionally healthy people, learning to adjust and cope with problems can lead to the related goal of self-development (Pardeck, 1993).

Self-actualization is a concept that is aligned with self-development. Self-development, similar to self-actualization, means the fullest, most complete differentiation and harmonious blending of all aspects of one's total well-being. Self-development means the psyche has evolved to a new center; that is, the self takes the place of the old center, the ego. The person who has achieved optimal self-development is similar to Jung's (1954) view of what human beings might evolve to once the process of self-actualization is complete. The self-actualized person is one who has fulfilled one's fullest potentials and has accepted the self (Pardeck, 1993).

Maslow (1971) provided another view of self-development through his concept of self-actualization. He felt humans have a drive to know the self better and to develop to their fullest potential. Maslow theorized that human nature is essentially good, and to strive for self-actualization is a positive process that leads people to reach their fullest potential. Maslow (1971) viewed most individuals as being in a constant state of striving to improve themselves; however, he believed very few people achieve the personal growth needed to become self-actualized. Most people are in a constant state of disequilibrium and are striving to resolve this state through self-development.

A self-actualized person displays high levels of all of the following characteristics: accepts self and others; seeks justice, order, truth, unity, and beauty; is able to solve problems; has a richness of emotional responses; has satisfying relationships with other people; and has a high sense of moral values.

Maslow felt that most psychologists study the stunted, crippled, and neurotic individuals, which ultimately results in a limited psychology. Thus, self-development and self-actualization have not received the emphasis needed within the field of psychology. Maslow emphasized focusing on emotionally healthy people rather than troubled ones; consequently, these two groups generate two types of theories—one aimed at growth and development and the other focused on pathology (Pardeck, 1993).

Presently, there are numerous self-help books offering strategies for enhancing self-actualization, which can enhance one's self-development. The titles included in Chapter 4 offer strategies to help one become more accepting of the self and others, to assist one in moving toward a problem-centered approach to life rather than a self-centered approach, and to increase one's creativity and resist conformity to the larger culture.

Some of the titles in Chapter 4 also deal with self-development issues that can become clinical problems if not resolved. These include such clinical problems as codependency, recovery from abuse, and chemical dependency. Other titles offer information for the healthy individual who wishes to enhance his or her self-development. The titles included in Chapter 4 can be used in individual treatment or in group settings.

SERIOUS ILLNESS

There are three basic models for understanding health: the disease, illness, and sickness models. The model used for defining health has a tremendous impact on the assessment and treatment process. For example, if one uses a disease model, health is viewed strictly in terms of the presence or absence of clearly identifiable physical signs and symptoms. If one approaches the issue of health from an illness model, one considers not only physical symptoms but also the psychosocial aspects of health. What constitutes health is strongly shaped by its definition and by the individual's subjective interpretation about one's own healthiness (Pardeck, 1996).

A disease model is based on the physical aspect of the individual. Disease is a biomedical concept that refers to the physiological features of nonhealth. A disease model for understanding health has numerous limitations. This approach continues to be the dominant model for the delivery of health care services in the United States (Pardeck and Yuen, 1997).

An illness approach to defining and understanding health is very different from the disease model. An illness can exist whether a disease is present or absent. If an individual defines the self as ill, even though physical symptoms are not present, an illness does exist. Even though an illness is often assumed to be caused by a disease, there is speculation that if one defines the self as ill, these subjective feelings can foster nonhealth (Pardeck, 1996).

The sickness model is based on the concepts of status, roles, and social identity. This model is grounded in the field of sociology and views health or the lack of health as being a label created by the larger society. The process of defining someone as sick can happen regardless of whether an illness or disease is present or not. Minuchin and Nichols (1993) focus their research on the psychosomatic aspect of sickness as defined by the family system.

Minuchin and Nichols (1993) stress that much of one's ability to cope with sickness or illness is affected by one's ability to adapt to his or her social environment. This means in a supportive social environment, individuals who have been labeled as sick will be better able to adapt and cope with disease and illness. Those social environments that are not supportive will result in poor adaptation for ill individuals (Kilpatrick and Holland, 1995).

The disease model appears to offer little for those who endorse self-help as an important tool for maintaining health and in treating disease or illness. The component that is lacking in the disease model is the social and subjective nature of health. Both of these aspects of health are dealt with far more effectively in the illness and sickness models (Pardeck, 1996).

Vega and Murphy (1990) argue that health is poorly understood using a pathological orientation, or disease model. They suggest that one should look to the client's culture or social environment, particularly the family system, in order to have a more holistic understanding of the concept of health. According to Vega and Murphy (1990), health is a highly relative issue that is influenced by genetics and one's subjective feelings about one's level of healthiness, as well as one's social environment.

Self-help plays an important role in the treatment of illness or sickness if one views these problems from psychosocial and societal perspectives. The self-help books presented in Chapter 4 largely reinforce a dynamic orientation for dealing with the concept of health. It must be noted that none of the works included deny the importance of the biological basis of disease or illness, but instead recognize the importance of defining health from a biological, psychological, and sociological perspective. Such a view offers a more holistic view of health that reinforces the active participation of the client in the assessment and treatment process.

SUBSTANCE-RELATED DISORDERS

Chemical dependency is best understood as the adaptive behavior of an individual embedded within a chemically dependent family system (Pardeck, 1993). Theorists increasingly agree with this position as an explanation for why family members abuse alcohol and other drugs (Gladding, 1995). There is clear evidence that the family system is critical to the initiation, maintenance, cessation, and prevention of alcohol and drug abuse (Kilpatrick and Holland, 1995).

A family systems approach suggests that individuals who abuse alcohol and drugs are significantly connected, both developmentally and physically, to their families (Pardeck, 1996). Their behavior is influenced by family interaction; when persons push for individuation and separation within the chemically dependent family system, the family resists the change. Codependent family systems attempt to retard or postpone the process of individuation, and this process results in dysfunctional family alignments (Pardeck, 1996). Often, children from chemically dependent systems continue these patterns of behavior into adulthood (Kilpatrick and Holland, 1995). Orton (1997) reports that at least eight million children in the United States live in alcoholic family systems. Wilson and Blocher (1990) found that sons of alcoholic fathers are five times more likely to become alcoholics, and daughters of alcoholic mothers are three times more likely to become alcoholics than children from nonalcoholic family systems.

Theorists maintain that chemical dependency is a family-based problem that affects and involves all family members (Gladding, 1995; Kilpatrick and Holland, 1995). Chemically dependent family systems tend to have rules that contribute to dysfunctional behaviors. For example, one rule is that the person affected by chemicals is the most important aspect of the family's life. The dependent person's top priority is abusing chemicals, whereas the family's priority is attempting to keep chemicals away from the dependent person. The priorities of the chemically dependent person and the family are in conflict (Pardeck, 1993).

Denial is also typical of the chemically dependent family system. Family members often do not see the chemical as the cause of the problem. Another rule is that the dependent person is not responsible for his or her behavior, a position that makes individual behavioral change difficult. At times, others are blamed for the person's behavior; thus, reality testing in the chemically dependent family system is limited. Family members in turn resist changing and feel more comfortable with the dependent family member abusing chemicals because this behavior maintains the dysfunctional family system. Unwritten rules also forbid talking about the chemical abuse, and, as with closed family systems in general, members resist outside intervention (Pardeck, 1993).

In the chemically dependent family system, all family members suffer from the chemical dependency, and each member plays a role in its maintenance. Thus, treatment of the chemically dependent family system involves each family member taking responsibility for his or her own behavior and helping the chemically dependent person recognize that he or she has a problem. Once this occurs, family treatment has a greater probability of success (Pardeck, 1993).

Factual information on the progression of chemical dependency is critical. There are clear cycles to the dependency process that must be stopped, and all family members are involved in this process. If the process is not altered, the chemically dependent individual will grow worse, and the family will become more pathological. Numerous self-help groups, which often use self-help books, are available for all members of the chemically dependent family system (Pardeck, 1996).

Chapter 4 offers self-help books that can help individuals and families confronted with chemical dependency. These books focus on codependency, children of alcoholics, teaching children about chemical dependency, and the neurochemical aspects of dependency. Many of the titles can be used as self-administered programs that can compliment one's recovery, and as titles recommended by the practitioner for the chemically dependent client and his or her family.

EXAMPLES OF BOOKS ON DIVORCE AND REMARRIAGE

The following offers an overview of quality books that focus on the problem of divorce. The examples of books on the topic of divorce covered in this chapter are representative of books that can be found in other clinical areas.

Dinosaurs Divorce: A Guide for Changing Families, by Brown and Brown (1986) is written for children ages three through eight who have experienced divorce. The book goes to the heart of problems common to children during and after divorce and offers advice for helping children deal with divorce. *Dinosaurs Divorce* is thirty pages long and has full-color pictures that illustrate the experiences of divorce in a family of dinosaurs.

Topics include why families experience divorce, what happens after divorce, how children feel during a divorce, what living in a one-parent family is like, and telling friends about the divorce. The book is basic and very easy for children to read and understand. Practitioners, children, and parents can read and discuss the examples in *Dinosaurs Divorce.* The book emphasizes the positive ways children can cope with the divorce process.

Gardner's (1983) *The Boys' and Girls' Book About Divorce* is an excellent self-help book. It discusses childhood fears and worries often common to children of divorce and is designed to help children face problems related to divorce. The work is for children over ten years of age. The book includes material based on the author's clinical practice with children of divorce. Gardner tells children not to blame themselves for the divorce and how to handle feelings of anger caused by the divorce.

Other topics include how children can get along with parents when living apart, problems related to playing one divorced parent against the other, ways of dealing with stepparents, and what to expect if a child must go to treatment because of problems related to divorce. This is one of the first books written specifically for children of divorce and continues to be used by many practitioners for helping children deal with divorce.

Gardner's (1977) other book on divorce, *The Parents' Book About Divorce,* provides advice to parents about how to tell children about divorce, how to help them deal with divorce, and approaches for helping children deal with issues following the divorce. Parents are advised of how to get counseling, cope with the demands of an ex-spouse, reduce guilt, and handle the emotions related to dating following a divorce.

This is an excellent book for parents exploring the many problems related to divorce. Practitioners will find the work particularly useful as an adjutant to counseling parents of divorce.

Kalter's (1990) *Growing Up with Divorce* is also for divorced parents and presents information to help them deal with emotional problems related to divorce. It is specifically designed to help parents counteract the long-term emotional problems that children may experience as a result of divorce. The book offers strategies to help children cope with the anger, confusion, and anxiety, in the present and future, related to the divorce. The author stresses that the reaction to divorce is related to the child's age and gender, and offers detailed experiences of children's reaction to divorce at various phases of the life cycle. This book is an excellent self-help book. Both children and parents of divorce will find the practical information included in the work helpful.

How It Feels When Parents Divorce, by Krementz (1984), presents nineteen girls and boys, ages eight to sixteen, who share their experiences and feelings related to the divorce experience. The children come from culturally diverse backgrounds. The title of each chapter is a child's name, includes a photo of the child, and his or her experiences with divorce. The children discuss changes in their lives, the confusion they felt when trying to cope with family breakdown, and the knowledge they gained because of the divorce.

This book is useful for children of divorce because it offers sincere commentaries that can be used by practitioners to help children cope with the divorce process. Parents of children of divorce will also find the work useful.

What Kind of Family Is This?, by Seuling (1985), focuses on a child who is attempting to resolve problems related to his parents divorce as he begins life in a blended family. The book is designed for children age four to six years.

Jeff is the central character of the story; Jeff's mom has remarried. After the remarriage, Jeff must move to a new house and learn to live with a new family. Jeff still loves his father and doesn't want another father. Jeff and his stepbrother even divide the bedroom in half but later decide to fix up the room together. Jeff finds it just takes time to get used to his new blended family.

A Case Example

The following case example illustrates the bibliotherapeutic process. The book used as a part of the treatment process is Seuling's (1985) *What Kind of Family Is This?* The client, eight-year-old John, began having problems with his schoolwork. The child appeared to be distraught and had problems interacting with other youngsters. John's teacher referred him to the school social worker; the social worker decided John could benefit from counseling. The social worker decided to use bibliotherapy as a part of the therapeutic process. After the first interview, the social worker found John lacked confidence in himself. The social worker noted the following comments John made during the interview, "I just can't do my school work," and "I am not smart enough to do good in school." The social worker also discovered John's parents had divorced when he was six. John's mother recently remarried, and John was having problems adjusting to his new blended family.

The social worker decided that the most pressing issue was to help John deal with the divorce of his parents. It was assumed that if he came to terms with the divorce, his other problems related to school work and interaction with other youngsters would improve.

During a counseling session, the social worker introduced John to the book entitled *What Kind of Family Is This?,* by Barbara Seuling (1985). The social worker read the book aloud to the John. As noted previously, this book is about a child named Jeff whose mother had recently remarried. Jeff must deal with many complex adjustment issues. In the end, Jeff finds it just takes time to get used to his new blended family.

Even though two years had passed since John's parents divorced, John was able to identify with the story's main character, Jeff. The social worker had John dictate a letter to her about how the story character felt about moving to a new blended family. This process provided insight into John's own feelings about his parents' divorce and his new blended family. After a number of treatment sessions, John gradually began to accept his parents' divorce and his new family. John also began to gain confidence in himself, and his schoolwork improved as did his interaction with others.

CONCLUSION

Books are widely used in treatment by psychologists, health care professionals, and others professionals. Evidence suggests that many laypersons use books to deal with issues related to personal growth and development. Even though the verdict is still out on the effectiveness of books in therapy, there is little to suggest that the popularity of bibliotherapy among professionals and laypersons will abate (Pardeck, 1993).

A number of psychologists have reacted negatively to increasing use of books in treatment (Starker, 1988). However, it would clearly be very difficult to regulate what is produced by the self-help book industry in a free society. What is important, however, is that consumers of self-help books and related reading materials, such as fiction, realize the limitations of bibliotherapy and that it is not a cure-all for problems (Pardeck and Pardeck, 1996). Therapists should only use books in treatment in a responsible fashion and continue to conduct research on the effectiveness of bibliotherapy in practice.

Even though books are widely used by both professionals and laypersons as a treatment tool, one must be aware of the limitations of the bibliotherapeutic approach (Pardeck and Pardeck, 1986). Rubin (1978) concludes the most important issue concerning the use of books in treatment is not necessarily what books do to people but rather what people do while reading books. In other words, a reader may develop unrealistic expectations about solving a problem through a book because the person does not know the limitations of bibliotherapy. Furthermore, the reader may misinterpret, noncomply, project into, or otherwise misuse books, and avoid dealing responsibly with a presenting problem (Giblin, 1989).

Practitioners should be particularly aware that if books are introduced in treatment at an inappropriate time, the chance of successful treatment is decreased. Bibliotherapy is most effective after a trusting relationship has been established between client and therapist. If a client is moving toward a speedy resolution of a presenting problem, there is little need for books in treatment. It should also be noted that books should not be employed as a single helping strategy but should be seen largely as an adjunct to treatment (Pardeck, 1993).

A critical issue related to books in treatment, both fiction and nonfiction, is the client's habit of reading; this is especially important when using bibliotherapy with children. It should be realized, however, that many books are on audiotape; thus the problem of the nonreader is less critical if a book is in an audio format. One must realize the bibliotherapeutic technique has generally been found more effective with clients whose reading abilities are average or above (Zaccaria and Moses, 1968). The therapist must also be aware of the reading and interest levels of the client, regardless of age. Reading that does not interest the client will not be helpful to the client. Finally, one must keep the above points in mind when using books as a tool in treatment. If the limitations of fiction and nonfiction self-help books are understood, the benefits of the bibliotherapeutic process can be realized by all who use books as a tool to help clients deal with problems.

Chapter 4

Useful Books for Clinical Intervention

This chapter provides practitioners with readily available information on fiction and nonfiction books that can be effectively used to treat various clinical problems. The books presented in this chapter may also be useful for those who simply wish to gain greater insight into a problem area and for others who wish to explore the reading materials available on various clinical problems.

Books offered in this chapter are grouped under clinical topics that include divorce and remarriage, dysfunctional families, parenting, self-development, serious illness, and substance-related disorders. There are over three hundred annotated books presented in this chapter that deal with these problem areas. The books are written for adults and children.

COVERAGE AND SCOPE

The majority of books annotated in this chapter were published in the 1980s to the present; a limited number of the books are from earlier time periods. The general criteria used for book selection included the following:

1. The book had to focus on one or more of the clinical topics covered in the work.
2. The book had to offer useful content on the problem area covered.
3. The book had to be clearly appropriate to the implementation of the bibliotherapeutic process.

Each book has an interest level (IL) indicated by age. If the interest level of the book is over eighteen years of age, the IL is followed by the word Adult. The reader will be able to gain insight into a book's content through the work's annotation. The annotation also provides enough information to allow the reader to be able to judge if a work is fiction or nonfiction.

ENTRIES

The annotated entries are arranged in alphabetical order by the author's last name. Many of the annotated works focus on more than one clinical problem. However, the primary clinical problem covered in a given work determined the problem area under which it was included. For example, a book on family dysfunction may include some content on chemical dependency. If the primary focus is on family dysfunction, however, the book was placed in that topic area.

INDEXES

The Author Index is a guide to the individuals who wrote the books annotated in each problem area in the chapter. The Title Index helps the reader locate a particular title. The numbers following the authors and titles in these two indexes refer to the books' main entry numbers within each of the problem areas. A Subject Index allows the reader to refer to specific subjects covered in the annotated entries. Like the two other indexes, the Subject Index refers the reader to the appropriate entry numbers within the chapter.

DIVORCE AND REMARRIAGE

1. Arendell, Terry. *Mothers and Divorce: Legal, Economic, and Social Dilemmas.* Berkeley: University of California Press, 1986.
   - This work explores the numerous issues related to divorce, including legal and economic. The author bases the book on an empirical study of the problem of divorce. IL: Adult

2. Belli, Melvin M., and Drantzler, Mel. *Divorcing.* New York: St. Martin's Press, 1990.
   - This book is written by a family therapist and an attorney. Discusses the legal and emotional problems associated with divorce. IL: Adult
3. Berman, Claire. *Adult Children of Divorce Speak Out.* Minneapolis, MN: CompCare Publishers, 1992.
   - Insights are offered for children who are experiencing divorce. The work presents interviews with men and women of all ages that have experienced the divorce of their parents. The work includes insights into developing new relationships. IL: Adult
4. Berstein, Anne C. *Yours, Mine and Ours: How Families Change when Remarried Parents Have a Child Together.* New York: Macmillan Publishers, 1989.
   - This book is written by a family therapist. The work is based on a study of the dynamics of blended families. IL: Adult
5. Brown, Laurence, and Brown, Marc. *Dinosaurs Divorce: A Guide for Changing Families.* Boston: Atlantic Monthly Press, 1986.
   - This text attempts to get to the heart of the feelings and problems common to children during and after divorce. The authors offer practical advice to children. IL: Ages 4-6
6. Burt, Mala Schuster, and Burt, Roger B. *What's Special About Our Stepfamily.* New York: Dolphin Books, 1983.
   - This book stresses that divorce is never easy, nor is the establishment of a blended family. The authors present the unique problems of children in blended families. Included are fill-in-the-blank questions and other related activities for children to answer about blended families. IL: Ages 5-10
7. Clapp, Genevieve. *Divorce and New Beginnings: An Authoritative Guide to Recovery and Growth, Solo Parenting, and Stepfamilies.* New York: Wiley, 1992.
   - This is a self-help book on divorce. The legal, emotional, and economic effects of divorce are covered. Various kinds of

parenting are explored—part-time, single, and stepparenting. IL: Adult

8. Clubb, Angela. *Love in the Blended Family: Stepfamilies.* Deerfield Beach, FL: Health Communications, 1991.

   - The author presents a view of the blended family from the perspective of the stepmother. The work focuses on a family configuration that includes children from the husband's prior marriage and two additional children born into the blended family. The theme of this work is to present the unique problems and concerns parents, particularly women, have in this kind of family. IL: Adult

9. Diamond, Susan Arnsberg. *Helping Children of Divorce: A Handbook for Parents and Teachers.* New York: Schocken Press, 1985.

   - This book is for parents and teachers who work with children experiencing divorce. The focus of the work is on helping children deal with common psychological and social problems related to divorce. IL: Adult

10. Dinkmeyer, Don, McKay, Gary, and McKay, Joyce L. *New Beginnings: Skills for Single Parents and Stepfamily Parents.* Champaign, IL: Research Press, 1987.

    - This manual presents new skills and ideas that focus on the needs of today's single and stepfamily parents. Case examples and illustrations are presented. Contents include self-esteem, relationship and behavior, personality, and emotional development. IL: Adult

11. Drescher, Joan. *My Mother's Getting Married.* New York: Dial Press, 1986.

    - This picture-book describes a common occurrence in today's society—remarriage of parents. The child in the book resents the parent's remarriage. IL: Ages 5-10

12. Eckler, James. *Step-by-Stepparenting: A Guide to Successful Living with a Blended Family.* White Hall, VA: Betterway Publications, 1988.

- This work covers the unique problems and concerns parents have in blended families. A variety of issues are covered including the games stepchildren play, the rights of the stepparent, name changes, the pros and cons of adoption, discipline, stepsibling rivalries, marital communication, grandparents, and dealing with the emotional and social development of children. IL: Adult

13. Einstein, Elizabeth, and Albert, Linda. *Strengthen Your Stepfamily.* Circle Pines, MN: American Guidance Service, 1986.

- The authors explore five major themes in their work: (1) how the structure of the stepfamily differs from other family structures; (2) couple relationships and how to communicate more effectively; (3) strategies for creating positive relationships; (4) children's feelings and behaviors in stepfamilies; and (5) approaches for helping stepfamilies function well. A number of exercises are included that can help stepfamilies improve social interaction. IL: Adult

14. Felker, Evelyn H. *Raising Other People's Kids.* Grand Rapids, MI: William B. Eermans Publishing, 1981.

- This work covers the struggle of raising nonbiological children. The author guides stepparents through a series of practical activities that help them improve their role as stepparents. IL: Adult

15. Francke, Linda Bird. *Growing Up Divorced.* New York: Check Fawcett Publishers, 1984.

- This book is based on interviews with children of divorced parents, and offers insights into the social and psychological effects of divorce. IL: Adult

16. Gardner, Richard. *The Boys' and Girls' Book About Divorce.* Northvale, NJ: Jason Aronson, 1970.

- This title discusses the childhood fears and worries common to children of divorce. It is designed to help children face problems related to divorce. The book includes material based on the author's clinical practice with children of divorce. Gardner tells children not to blame themselves for the divorce and how to handle feelings of anger caused by the divorce. IL: Ages 10-18

17. Gardner, Richard. *The Parents' Book About Divorce.* New York: Doubleday, 1977.
    - Provides advice to parents about how to tell children about divorce, how to help them deal with divorce, and approaches for helping children deal with issues following the divorce. Parents are advised on how to seek counseling, cope with the demands of an ex-spouse, reduce guilt, and handle the emotions related to dating following a divorce. IL: Adult
18. Janda, Louis, and MacCormack, Ellen. *The Second Time Around: Why Some Second Marriages Fail.* New York: Carol Publishing, 1991.
    - The work focuses on a variety of issues related to stepfamilies. The authors base their writing on case studies of over one hundred people who were in second marriages. The reader learns about the issues related to blended families through case studies. Even though a number of blended families fail, the authors stress that many couples do find the love, trust, and security they did not experience in first marriages. IL: Adult
19. Kalter, Neil. *Growing Up with Divorce.* New York: The Free Press, 1990.
    - This book is for divorced parents and presents information to help them deal with emotional problems related to divorce. It is specifically designed to help parents counteract the long-term emotional problems that children may experience as a result of divorce. The book offers strategies to help children cope with the anger, confusion, and anxiety related to divorce in the present and future. IL: Adult
20. Keshet, Jamie K. *Love and Power in the Stepfamily: A Practical Guide.* New York: McGraw-Hill, 1987.
    - This book includes information on all aspects of creating blended families. Topics include discussions on parenting after divorce, introducing children to new partners, affection

and unification, remarried couples, and the new baby. IL: Adult

21. Krantzler, Mel. *Learning to Love Again.* New York: Harper and Row Publishers, 1987.

    - This book analyzes the development of new relationships when old ones have failed. Particular emphasis on new living arrangements, creating new commitments, and stepchildren. IL: Adult

22. Krementz, Jill. *How It Feels When Parents Divorce.* New York: Knopf, 1984.

    - Nineteen boys and girls share the experiences and feelings they had while adjusting to divorced families. The children represent several ethnic groups and a wide range of experiences, ranging from a background of violence in the home to resolution of friendly joint custody. IL: Ages 11-14

23. Pogue, Carolyn. *The Weekend Parent: Learning to Live Without Full-Time Kids.* Minneapolis: CompCare Publishers, 1992.

    - This work addresses sensitive issues related to loss or surrender of child custody. These are the personal stories of twenty men and women who have lost custody and subsequently discovered new roles noncustodial parents can play in the lives of their children. IL: Adult

24. Rosin, Mark. *Step-Fathering.* New York: Simon and Schuster, 1987.

    - This book offers advice for stepfathers in blended families. The author basis this advice on in-depth interviews with over fifty stepfathers. Topics include the following: problems related to combining families; discipline and authority within stepfamilies; communication issues related to blended families; and the strengths and rewards of stepparenting. IL: Adult

25. Sandvig, Karen J. *Adult Children of Divorce: Haunting Problems and Healthy Solutions.* Waco, TX: Word, Inc., 1990.

    - Based on exhaustive research and real-life examples (loneliness, low self-esteem, and others), this book shows how to break the cycle and keep these feelings from contributing to dysfunctional relationships a generation after a divorce. IL: Adult

26. Seuling, Barbara. *What Kind of Family Is This?* Racine, WI: Western Publishing, 1985.
    - Focuses on a child who is attempting to resolve problems related to his parents' divorce as he begins life in a blended family. Jeff is the central character of the story; Jeff's mom has remarried. After the remarriage, Jeff must move to a new house and learn to live with a new family. Jeff still loves his father and does not want another father. Jeff and his step-brother even divide the bedroom in half, but later decide to fix up the room together. Jeff finds it just takes time to get use to his new blended family. IL: Ages 4-6
27. Visher, Emily, and Visher, John. *Old Loyalties, New Ties: Therapeutic Strategies with Stepfamilies.* New York: Brunner/Mazel, 1988.
    - A broad range of topics are covered to help stepfamilies cope more effectively. The book discusses how therapy for remarried families differs from therapy for other kinds of family systems. One of the core issues in the work is the problem of how loyalties to a previous family system impact the blended family. The authors outline the therapeutic strategies they believe are most effective with stepfamilies. Many case studies are offered throughout the book that illustrate the authors' therapeutic approach. IL: Adult
28. Visher, Emily, and Visher, John. *How to Win as a Stepfamily.* New York: Drmbner Books, 1982.
    - The emphasis of this work is on the process of creating blended families. Included are chapters on forming new relationships, dealing with former spouses, understanding legal issues, and helping children adjust to the blended family. IL: Adult
29. Wallerstein, Judith, and Blakeslee, Sandra. *Second Chances: Men, Women and Children a Decade After Divorce.* New York: Ticknor and Fields, 1989.

- This book presents the economic and psychological effects of divorce on children. The work is based on a study of sixty middle-class divorced families. IL: Adult

DYSFUNCTIONAL FAMILIES

30. Adams, Kenneth M. *Silently Seduced: When Parents Make Their Children Partners—Understanding Covert Incest.* Deerfield Beach, FL: Health Communications, Inc., 1991.
    - The focus of this work is on the serious social problem of incest. The work provides incest victims with information on how their lives continue to be affected after the incest has stopped and how to begin the process of recovery. IL: Adult
31. Adler, C. S. *Fly Free.* New Jersey: Coward-McCann, 1984.
    - Shari learns to cope with having been abused. She continues to live with her mother even though their relationship is strained. IL: Ages 6-8
32. Amber. *Please Say You're Sorry.* Minneapolis: CompCare Publishers, 1992.
    - This work is designed for women who have survived incest. Through handwritten and self-illustrated testimony, the author shares her own story concerning victimization. IL: Adult
33. Anderson, Deborah, and Finne, Martha. *Margaret's Story.* Minneapolis: Dillion Press, 1986.
    - Margaret must go to court because she has been sexually abused. Margaret was afraid to tell her parents because the perpetrator told her not to tell anyone. Margaret finds out that what happened to her is against the law. This book is based on an actual case. IL: Ages 5-10
34. Anderson, Deborah, and Finne, Martha. *Michael's Story.* Minneapolis: Dillion Press, 1986.
    - Michael's parents make him feel bad about himself. His mother tells him that he is fat and his dad calls him stupid.

After a fight at school, Michael talks to a social worker. Therapy helps him deal with his sadness and anger. IL: Ages 5-10

35. Anderson, Deborah, and Finne, Martha. *Robin's Story.* Minneapolis: Dillion Press, 1986.
    - Robin's mother often gets mad and spanks him. She spanks him with a belt and cuts him with a cookie tin thrown at him. He must go to a physician because of the injury, and the past physical abuse is discovered. IL: Ages 5-8
36. Baker, Sally A. *Family Violence and the Chemical Connection.* Deerfield Beach, FL: Health Communications, Inc., 1992.
    - The author illustrates the relationship between chemical abuse and family violence. The work claims that family violence is a common problem, and strategies are presented for dealing with the problems associated with family violence. IL: Adult
37. Bass, Ellen, and Davis, Laura. *The Courage to Heal: A Guide for Women of Child Sexual Abuse.* New York: HarperCollins Publishers, Inc., 1988.
    - The goal of this book is to empower survivors of childhood sexual abuse. Various strategies are presented to help survivors deal with the aftermath of this serious social problem. IL: Adult
38. Bass, Ellen, and Thorton, Louise, (eds). *I Never Told Anyone: Writings by Women Survivors of Child Abuse.* New York: HarperCollins Publishers, Inc., 1991.
    - This work offers testimonies from suvivors of childhood sexual abuse. A list of resource groups and treatment centers for treating child abuse is included. IL: Adult
39. Bradshaw, John. *Healing the Shame That Binds You.* Deerfield Beach, FL: Health Communications, 1988.
    - The focus of this book is on toxic shame. Toxic shame is present in individuals who feel that things are helpless and that they are worthless. Individuals with toxic shame feel they lack control and power over their lives. According to the author, toxic shame is created during childhood. IL: Adult

40. Byars, Betsy. *Cracker Jackson.* New York: Viking, 1984.

    • An eleven-year-year-old boy is instrumental in getting his ex-babysitter to seek shelter from her husband, who beats her and their baby. IL: Ages 10-13

41. Byars, Betsy. *The Pinballs.* New York: Harper and Row, 1977.

    • Three foster children—two teenagers who have been physically abused and a young boy abandoned by his mother—share a home. They share feelings about being victims of abuse and begin to feel like a family within the security of their foster home. IL: Ages 11-16

42. Davis, Laura. *Allies in Healing: When the Person You Love Was Sexually Abused as a Child.* New York: HarperCollins Publishers, Inc., 1991.

    • This work addresses the needs of partners and spouses of survivors of childhood sexual abuse. Various strategies are offered to deal with this serious social problem. IL: Adult

43. Davis, Laura. *The Courage to Heal Workbook: For Women and Men Survivors of Child Sexual Abuse.* New York: HarperCollins Publishers, Inc., 1990.

    • This book is designed to help those who were victims of child abuse. It offers a combination of checklists, writing exercises, art projects, and activities that offer a step-by-step guide to the healing process. IL: Adult

44. Girard, Linda. *My Body Is Private.* Niles, IL: Albert Whitman and Company, 1984.

    • This book discusses appropriate and inappropriate touching of children by adults. In the language of a child, the book addresses the parts of the child's body that should or should not be touched by adults, unless there is good reason. The book explains to children what they should do if an adult touches private parts of the child's body. Jon R. Conte, PhD, includes a note to parents about what they should do if a child is sexually abused, including how to contact a child protection agency. IL: Ages 5-10

45. Graber, Ken. *Ghosts in the Bedroom: A Guide for Partners of Incest Survivors.* Deerfield Beach, FL: Health Communications, Inc., 1991.

    - This work presents a step-by-step guide to comfort and guide partners of incest survivors. Various insights and activities are included to accomplish this goal. IL: Adult

46. Haskins, James. *The Child Abuse Help Book.* Niles, IL: Albert Whitman, 1981.

    - In this book, the problems that lead to and stem from child abuse accompany directions for help, including a list of agencies and resource centers, and suggestions for personal action. IL: Ages 11-14

47. Holland, Ruth. *Mill Child.* New York: Macmillan, 1970.

    - A history of child labor in factories and mines reveals the exploitation and abuse of migrant children that continues today. IL: Ages 11-14.

48. Hunt, Irene. *The Lottery Rose.* New York: Charles Scribner's, 1976.

    - Physically abused by his alcoholic mother and her boyfriend, a seven-year-old boy has behavioral problems and becomes distrustful and isolated from others. He is reluctant to enter a boy's home, but only there does he develop a positive relationship with other adults and counselors. IL: Ages 5-10

49. Hunter, Mic. *Abused Boys: The Neglected Victims of Sexual Abuse.* Minneapolis: CompCare Publishers, 1989.

    - Each year thousands of boys are sexually abused. Often, later in life, these children have difficulty achieving intimacy with their partners. The author attempts to offer help and healing for adults recovering from child maltreatment. A number of first-person stories are presented, and an extensive resource guide is also offered. IL: Adult

50. Hyde, Margaret O. *Cry Softly! The Story of Child Abuse.* Philadelphia: Westminster, 1980.

- This story offers an easy-to-read overview of historical and contemporary patterns of child abuse, with a listing of organizations for obtaining help. IL: Ages 10-13

51. Kellogg, Marjorie. *Like the Lion's Tooth.* New York: Farrar, Straus, and Giroux, 1972.

- Eleven-year-old Ben, who has been physically and sexually abused by his father, is sent to a school for "problem children." He runs away from the school in an attempt to find his mother. Finally, Ben resigns himself to his situation and begins making friends. IL: Ages 11-14

52. Lew, Mike. *Victims No Longer: Men Recovering from Incest and Other Sexual Child Abuse.* Minneapolis: CompCare Publishers, 1990.

- The author suggests that our culture has no room for male victims of child abuse. Often male victims are expected to deal with the problem of incest on their own; that is, to deal with it like a man. The work seeks to dismiss this myth, and to help male victims deal with the denial, grief, loss, anger, and other issues that result from sexual abuse. IL: Adult

53. MacPherson, Margaret. *The Rough Road.* San Diego: Harcourt Brace Jovanovich, 1966.

- A child who is mistreated by his foster parents has little joy in life. He is able to improve his emotional well-being after he makes a close friendship with someone who cares. IL: Ages 11-14

54. Maltz, Wendy. *The Sexual Healing Journey: A Guide for Survivors of Sexual Abuse.* New York: HarperCollins, 1991.

- This is a how-to, personal therapy book that offers a number of cases on the problems associated with those who have survived sexual abuse. The author stresses that abuse may become buried in a victim's unconscious self and thus contribute to sexual dysfunction. The work discusses what constitutes sexual abuse and the myths that surround this serious social problem. IL: Adult

55. Martin, Del. *Battered Wives.* Volcano, CA: Volcano Press, 1981.

    - This book is designed for women who have been in an abusive relationship or who continue to live in such a relationship. The work is designed for all women. The author feels battering is caused by the negative attitudes toward women in society and not necessarily the interaction between men and women. The work offers insight into the problem of battering. IL: Adult

56. Mazer, Harry. *The War on Villa Street.* New York: Delacort, 1978.

    - Willis, an eight-year-old boy, is frequently beaten by his alcoholic father—once to a point near unconsciousness. After striking back at his father, Willis runs away but returns hoping things will improve. IL: Ages 11-14

57. Moeri, Louise. *The Girl Who Lived on the Ferris Wheel.* New York: Avon, 1979.

    - In a disturbing and suspenseful book, a girl's emotionally troubled mother beats her. The girl reports the mother to the authorities. IL: Ages 10-14

58. Napier, Augustus, and Whitaker, Carl. *The Family Crucible.* New York: Harper and Row, 1978.

    - The work presents a family systems approach to solving family problems. The authors are leading family therapists who have contributed a great deal to the field. They describe in some detail the systems orientation and how this theory applies to family therapy. A basic premise of the book is that most problems that seem to be the property of a single individual actually evolved from relationships within the family. IL: Adult

59. Nestingen, Signe, and Lewis, Laurel. *Growing Beyond Abuse.* Minneapolis: CompCare Publishers, 1991.

    - This is a workbook for survivors of sexual exploitation and childhood sexual abuse. The work offers poetry and prose, healing reading, and written exercises to help individuals deal with the pain of victimization. IL: Adult

60. Newman, Susan. *Never Say Yes to a Stranger: What Every Child Should Know to Stay Safe.* New York: Putnam/Perigee, 1985.

    • This book teaches children to have a healthy fear of strangers and discusses what children should do when they find themselves in trouble with a stranger. IL: Ages 4-10

61. NiCarthy, Ginny, and Davidson, Sue. *You Can Be Free: An Easy-to-Read Handbook for Abused Women.* Minneapolis: CompCare Publishers, 1989.

    • This book presents basic insights into the problems of women who have been victims of abuse. The author attempts to offer support, answers, and actions that women can take when they are being abused by someone they love. IL: Adult

62. NiCarthy, Ginny. *Getting Free: You Can End Abuse and Take Back Your Life,* second edition. Seattle: The Seal Press, 1986.

    • This book is based on the experiences of the author working with battered women. The work is divided into six parts: (1) making the decision to leave or stay; (2) getting professional help; (3) helping yourself to survival; (4) after you leave; (5) the ones who got away; and (6) new directions. The author includes a national survey that provides information from abused women. A number of exercises are included to help battered women in their recovery from abuse. IL: Adult

63. O'Hanlon, Jacklyn. *Fair Game.* New York: Dial Press, 1977.

    • Fourteen-year-old Denise is in turmoil after she discovers her new stepfather watching her undress. When her stepfather makes sexual advances toward Denise's younger sister and a friend, the girls tell Denise's mother, who forces her husband to leave. IL: Ages 11-18

64. Orr, Rebecca. *Gunner's Run.* New York: Harper and Row, 1980.

    • Frequently beaten by his alcoholic father, nine-year-old Gunner runs away from home. He is able to develop a better self-concept through his association with an elderly man who is dying. IL: Ages 8-11

65. Ratner, Ellen. *The Other Side of the Family: A Book for Recovery from Abuse, Incest, and Neglect.* Deerfield Beach, FL: Health Communications, Inc., 1990.

    - The issues related to surviving child maltreatment are presented. Offered are treatment strategies for combating the problem of victimization. IL: Adult

66. Roberts, Willo. *Don't Hurt Laurie.* New York: Atheneum, 1978.

    - Physically abused by her mother since the age of three, eleven-year old Laurie is afraid to approach any adult about the situation. With the aid of her concerned stepbrother, Laurie is finally able to tell her stepfather the truth, after which her mother eventually receives treatment. IL: Ages 11-14

67. Smith, Doris. *Tough Chauncey.* New York: Morrow, 1974.

    - A boy is caught between torrents of physical and verbal abuse from his dictatorial grandfather. The child's mother does not show him affection, and foster care finally appears to be the best placement for the boy. IL: Ages 11-14

68. Stanek, Muriel. *Don't Hurt Me, Mama.* Niles, IL: Whitman, 1983.

    - A girl narrates the story of how her mother begins neglecting and abusing her until school officials intervene. The child receives help from social services and a community mental health center. IL: Ages 5-8

69. Wachter, Oralee. *Close to Home.* New York: Scholastic, 1986.

    - The book addresses various child-safety issues in a nonthreatening manner. A number of abduction situations are portrayed. IL: Ages 8-11

70. Walker, Lenore. *The Battered Woman.* New York: Harper and Row, 1979.

    - This work is divided into three main parts. Part I covers the psychology of the battered woman; the myths and realities of abuse are offered. Part II provides information on the experiences of battered women. Problems confronting battered women in the legal and medical systems are covered in Part

III. This work offers a number of helpful exercises to assist women in dealing with the psychological pain resulting from battering. IL: Adult

71. Wolter, Dwight Lee. *My Child, My Teacher, My Friend: One Man's View of Parenting in Recovery.* Minneapolis: CompCare Publishers, 1991.

   - This work is intended for all parents in recovery, particularly single parents and those who grew up in dysfunctional families. Practical help and wisdom concerning family dysfunction are presented. IL: Adult

PARENTING

72. Baldwin, Rahima. *You Are Your Child's First Teacher.* Berkeley: Celestial Arts, 1989.

   - This book stresses the numerous approaches offered on how to parent your children. The author offers a new way of understanding the human being so that parents can be better parents. The work is based on the Montessori theoretical approach. IL: Adult

73. Blechman, Elaine A. *Solving Child Behavior Problems at Home and at School.* Champaign, IL: Research Press, 1985.

   - This book provides step-by-step methods for improving children's behavior. It includes guidelines to help prevent common behavior problems from escalating into more serious ones. IL: Adult

74. Brazelton, T. Berry. *Touchpoint.* Reading, MA: Addison-Wesley, 1992.

   - This parenting self-help book covers all phases of child development. Unlike many self-help books on parenting, it stresses the special role of fathers and other socializing agents in children's development. These other agents include grandparents and other caregivers. IL: Adult

75. Brazelton, T. Berry. *Infants and Mothers.* New York: Delta/Seymour Lawrence, 1983.

- The work describes infant temperament and developmental milestones in the first year of life. This is a self-help book designed for parents. It focuses on three different types of temperament styles in infants: active baby, average baby, and quiet baby. The work concludes that parents should be sensitive observers of their baby's temperament and behavior. This sensitivity will help parents chart parenting strategies that meet the needs of their children. IL: Adult

76. Brazelton, T. Berry. *What Every Baby Knows.* Reading, MA: Addison-Wesley, 1987.

- A broad approach is offered based on the experiences of five different families. The author offers analyses of the five families in the areas of child rearing, discipline, fears, sibling rivalry, separation and divorce, and other related areas. The author presents some of the most important aspects of being an effective and competent parent. IL: Adult

77. Brondino, Jeanne; Brann, Shellie; Coatsworth, Scott; Sonzeno, Heidi; Swain, Cheryl, and Tulao, Frances. *Raising Each Other: A Book for Teens and Parents.* Minneapolis: Comp-Care Publishers, 1990.

- This book is taken directly from real-life exchanges between parents and high school students. In this work, parents and teens share their perspectives on issues of freedom, privacy, trust, responsibility, money, sex, and religion. IL: Adult

78. Canter, Lee, and Canter, Marlene. *Assertive Discipline for Parents.* New York: HarperCollins Publishers, Inc., 1988.

- This is a guide to enable parents to use new approaches to raising their children. The work offers strategies for helping parents not to be manipulated by their children and to use positive support when children behave. IL: Adult

79. Caplan, Frank. *The First Twelve Months of Life.* New York: Bantam, 1973.

- The first year of life is the focus of this book. A month-by-month assessment of normal infant development is presented. Feeding, language, sleeping, and parental emotions are examples of topics covered in the work. Each chapter offers a developmental chart outlining the appropriate sensory, motor, language, mental, and social development milestones for each month. IL: Adult

80. Caron, Ann F. *Don't Stop Loving Me: A Reassuring Guide for Mothers of Adolescent Daughters.* New York: HarperCollins Publishers, Inc., 1992.

   - The author explores the issues that affect mothers and daughters, including trust, dependency, sex, peers, friends, competition, drug use, and discipline. The work illustrates the ups and downs of mothers and their adolescent daughters. IL: Adult

81. Comer, James P., and Poussaint, Alvin E. *Raising Black Children.* New York: Plume, 1992.

   - This book argues that parents raising minority children face additional difficulties not faced by other parents. The author recommends ways the parents can improve the self-esteem and identity of minority children and offers suggestions to confront racism. The book uses a question and answer format for teaching the special needs of black children. IL: Adult

82. Dinkmeyer, Don, and McKay, Gary P. *Systematic Training for Effective Parenting.* Circle Pines, MN: American Guidance Service, 1990.

   - This work stresses an Adlerian model for effective parenting. It offers principles of logical consequences over punishment and of using cooperation versus power in the child-rearing process. IL: Adult

83. Dreikurs, Rudolph. *Children: The Challenge.* New York: Hawthorn Books, 1964.

   - The book is designed to help parents understand their children. The author offers techniques for responding to negative behaviors of children and appropriate strategies for disciplining children. The work is designed to improve parenting and the lives of children. IL: Adult

84. Dumont, Larry. *Surviving Adolescence: Helping Your Child Through the Struggle.* New York: Villard Books, 1991.

    - This book covers the problems and related issues that emerge during adolescence. The author attempts to educate the parent about the early-warning signs of adolescent problems ranging from drug abuse to learning disabilities. Suggested treatment strategies for troubled adolescents include counseling and group counseling. IL: Adult

85. Dunn, Judy, and Plomin, Robert . *Separate Lives: Why Siblings Are So Different.* New York: Basic Books, 1992.

    - The authors argue that the home environment plays a bigger role than genetic makeup in a child's development. The work is based on research on the topic of why siblings differ in their development. IL: Adult

86. Edelman, Marian Wright. *The Measure of Our Success: A Letter to My Children and Yours.* Boston: Beacon Press, 1992.

    - The author has been working for the advancement of children for several decades. The book stresses the fact that children represent the most important resource in our society and that they truly are the future. The book argues that the health and well-being of our nation's children and parents are critical to the survival of society. IL: Adult

87. Eisenber, Arlene, Murkoff, Heidi, and Hathaway, Nancy. *What to Expect the First Year.* New York: Workman, 1989.

    - The author offers a broad-based approach to infant development during the first year of life. The work is very long (over 600 pages) and offers facts and practical tips on how babies develop. Both medical and parenting advice is offered. IL: Adult

88. Elkind, David. *All Grown Up and No Place to Go: Teenagers in Crisis.* Reading, MA: Addison-Wesley, 1984.

    - This work concludes that parenting is more difficult now than ever before. The author suggests that teenagers are expected to confront adult challenges early in life and are being pressured into adult roles too soon. Teenagers' emotional needs are also neglected by the school system and the larger community. Approaches for improving the well-being of teenagers is offered in the book. IL: Adult

89. Elkind, David. *The Hurried Child: Growing Up Too Fast Too Soon.* Reading, MA: Addison-Wesley, 1988.

   - Here, Elkind describes the pervasive and harmful circumstances all too many children experience in American society. The author suggests that parents in today's society place too much pressure on children to grow up too soon. The excessive demands of parents on children can be found not only in academics but also in athletics. The book suggests that parents should respect the child's timetable for development. IL: Adult

90. Frances L., Bates Ames, Louise, and Baker, Sidney. *Child Behavior: The Classic Child Care Manual from the Gesell Institute of Human Behavior.* New York: HarperCollins Publishers, Inc., 1982.

   - This is a book that offers strategies for enhancing the lives of children and improving their behavior. It is designed for parents, teachers, and others who care for children. IL: Adult

91. Ginnot, Aim. *Between Parent and Teenager.* New York: Avon, 1969.

   - This work targets parents who wish to communicate more effectively with their teenagers. A number of basic strategies are outlined to help parents better understand and communicate with adolescents. The book covers the nature of the changes that take place during the adolescent years. A number of recommended approaches for handling conflict are presented. A wide range of examples illustrate how parents and teenagers can grow, learn, and change. IL: Adult

92. Gordon, Thomas. *Parenting Effectiveness Training.* New York: Wyden, 1970.

   - This work describes appropriate communication for parents when working with children. Problem-solving approaches are offered for improving the parenting process. IL: Adult

93. Guarendi, Ray. *Back to the Family: How to Encourage Traditional Values in Complicated Times.* New York: Basic Books, 1990.

    - This work describes the characteristics of the psychologically healthy family. The author is a specialist in the field of parenting and family issues. The book offers a how-to manual for parents who wish to improve family living; the manual is based on the author's research on and work with families. IL: Adult

94. Hart, Louise. *The Winning Family: Increasing Self-Esteem in Your Children and Yourself.* Deerfield Beach, FL: Health Communications, 1990.

    - This book provides specific, practical methods for developing communication and leadership skills in families. Includes discussion of skills needed for effective living, self-esteem, and mental health. IL: Adult

95. Leach, Penelope. *Babyhood,* second edition. New York: Alfred A. Knopf, 1983.

    - This book describes infant development from birth to age two. The author chronicles the physical, emotional, and mental development of babies during the first two years of life. Advice is offered for parents on a variety of developmental issues including feeding, sleeping, toilet training, mobility, language, and fears. IL: Adult

96. Nelson, Jane. *Positive Discipline,* second edition. New York: Ballantine, 1987.

    - This book is written for both parents and teachers; it is designed to help adults better understand children and discipline them so they can learn to be self-disciplined and responsible. The author recommends that parents should not overpunish children and should teach them logical consequences of misbehavior. The book is designed to offer positive discipline techniques that enable children to maintain their self-respect and understand that parents love and accept them. IL: Adult

97. Patterson, Gerald R. *Families: Applications of Social Learning to Family Life.* Champaign, IL: Research Press, 1975.
    - This work contains social learning procedures designed to bring about desired changes in the family unit. The author uses a program learning format that helps parents recognize the crucial role they play in shaping their children's behavior. IL: Adult
98. Patterson, Gerald R. *Living with Children: New Methods for Parents and Teachers.* Champaign, IL: Research Press, 1976.
    - This manual shows how children learn behavior and how they actually train parents to behave. It is written for parents and teachers who have little or no background in social learning theory. IL: Adult
99. Reaves, John, and Austin, James. *How to Find Help for a Troubled Kid.* New York: HarperCollins Publishers, Inc., 1991.
    - This book is designed for parents dealing with their troubled adolescents. The work covers topics such as teenage pregnancy, depression, mental illness, drug and alcohol abuse, and school problems. The index provides information on counseling hotlines, treatment centers, and drug and alcohol programs. IL: Adult
100. Salk, Lee. *Familyhood.* New York: Simon and Schuster, 1992.
    - This book is about the importance of families in children's development. The author emphasizes that the structure of families has changed enormously in recent years because of high divorce rates, increasing numbers of blended families, and the high numbers of families where both parents work. Even though the family has gone through significant changes, the values families cherish have not changed. This conclusion is based on extensive research the author conducted on a family values survey. The work should be helpful for parents who wish to instill positive values in their children. IL: Adult
101. Sanger, Sirgay, and Kelly, John. *The Woman Who Works, the Parent Who Cares.* New York: HarperCollins Publishers, Inc., 1992.

- A psychiatrist offers a program to demonstrate how the lifestyle of today's working woman can encourage the development of a more self-confident, independent, and socially developed child. IL: Adult

102. Schaefer, Charles E. *How to Talk to Children About Really Important Things.* New York: HarperCollins Publishers, Inc., 1992.

 - This work is designed to foster better communication between parents and their five- to ten-year-old children. The topics covered include going to the hospital, moving, understanding an alcoholic parent, death, abuse, divorce, prejudice, religion, and war. IL: Adult

103. Sifford, Darrell. *The Only Child: Being One, Loving One . . . Understanding One, Raising One.* New York: HarperCollins Publishers, Inc., 1990.

 - Only children are different and have unique needs. This book draws on case studies and interviews with psychologists and other helping professionals. The work is designed to help parents of only children. IL: Adult

104. Sloane, Howard N. *The Good Kid Book: How to Solve the 16 Most Common Behavior Problems.* Champaign, IL: Research Press, 1988.

 - This is a manual for parents who need help with specific child behavior problems. Each chapter is a self-contained behavior guide with step-by-step procedures for helping children overcome specific behavioral problems. IL: Adult

105. Smith, Judith M., and Smith, Donald E. P. *Child Management: A Program for Parents and Teachers.* Champaign, IL: Research Press, 1976.

 - This work illustrates how to help children learn appropriate behavior. The manual contains a programmed format. Values and morals training are offered. Examples of problem situations that teach children to consider the consequences of decision making are presented. IL: Adult

106. Spock, Benjamin, and Rothberg, Michael. *Dr. Spock's Baby and Child Care.* New York: E. P. Dutton, 1985.

   - This self-help book was initially published in 1945. It offers a broad approach to infant's and children's development. It has a great deal of medical advice that parents will find useful and also discusses child rearing. The book includes information on child abuse, neglect, and permissiveness. IL: Adult

107. Spock, Benjamin. *Dr. Spock on Parenting.* New York: Simon and Schuster, 1988.

   - The work emphasizes how to become a better parent and offers strategies for improving the social and emotional development of children. Topics covered in the book include anxieties, fathering, divorce, new baby, sleep problems, discipline, attitudes, health, and nutrition. The author stresses parents should provide structure to the lives of children in firm and clear ways. IL: Adult

108. Steinberg, Laurence, and Levine, Ann. *You and Your Adolescent: A Parent's Guide for Ages 10-19.* New York: HarperCollins Publishers, Inc., 1990.

   - This is a manual for parents raising adolescents. The work explores most of the major developmental crises confronting both parents and their adolescent children. IL: Adult

109. Wheelan, Susan A., and Silberman, Melvin L. *How to Discipline Without Feeling Guilty: Assertive Relationships with Children.* Champaign, IL: Research Press, 1980.

   - This is a guide for helping parents and teachers evaluate their relationships with children. It highlights the similarities and differences between parenting and teaching while it addresses the specific needs of both. Examples illustrate the techniques for disciplining children. IL: Adult

110. White, Burton. *The First Three Years of Life.* New York: Prentice-Hall Press, 1985.

   - This work is designed for parents of infants and young children. The author provides an in-depth discussion of motor, sensory, emotional, sociabilty, and language milestones during the first three years of life. Recommended and nonrecommended parenting practices are presented. The recommended practices are designed to help every child reach his or her maximum level of competence. IL: Adult

111. Zarrow, Teryl. *The Mother Side of Midnight.* Reading, MA: Addison-Wesley, 1992.

   • The struggles and rewards of parenting are discussed. Familiar parenting activities are covered; these include mealtime, family activities, birthday parties, and caring for pets. The author offers parenting situations with which the reader can identify. IL: Adult

112. Zionst, Paul, and Simpson, Richard L. *Understanding Children and Youth with Emotional and Behavioral Problems: A Handbook for Parents and Professionals.* Austin, TX: Pro-Ed, 1990.

   • This work is designed for parents, families, and professionals. The goal of the book is to further one's understanding of troubled children and the services available to meet their needs. It provides straightforward, basic information about childhood and adolescent emotional and behavioral problems. IL: Adult

Adoption

113. Anderson, C. W. *Lonesome Little Colt.* New York: Macmillan, 1974.

   • After a colt's mother dies, he is lonely and frightened. His colt friends all have mothers they can run to. A new mare brought to the farm adopts the little colt. IL: Ages 5-8

114. Arms, Suzanne. *Adoption: A Handful of Hope.* Berkeley, CA: Celestial Arts, 1989.

   • This work contains a series of case studies that offer the personal and moving accounts of children who have been adopted, adoptive parents, and women who have given their babies for adoption. The author attempts to show how the process of adoption can be improved for all parties involved. IL: Adult

115. Bates, Betty. *It Must've Been the Fish Sticks.* New York: Holiday House, 1982.
    - Brian discovers that his biological mother is alive. He confronts his parents and is eventually taken to Ohio to visit his biological mother. This book focuses on conflicting loyalties. IL: Ages 10-13
116. Bawden, Nina. *The Finding.* New York: Lothrop, 1985.
    - Alex is placed in an adoptive family. Alex feels loved and secure in his family but runs off because of a crisis. The crisis resolved, and Alex returns to his adoptive family. IL: Ages 9-12
117. Bloomquist, Geraldine M., and Bloomquist, Paul B. *Zachary's New Home.* New York: Magination Press, 1990.
    - This book is written for children entering adoption or foster care. The book deals with feelings through animal characters. IL: Ages 3-8
118. Blume, Judy. *Just as Long as We're Together.* New York: Orchard, 1987.
    - Three preadolescent girls face problems related to friendship, growing up, parental separation, fears of nuclear war, and placement for adoption. One of the girls, Alison, is a Korean girl who has been adopted. Alison's adoptive family is expecting a baby, and Alison is afraid her family won't want her anymore because she is adopted. IL: Ages 11-18
119. Brodzinsky, Anne. *The Mulberry Bird: A Story of an Adoption.* Indianapolis, IN: Perspective Press, 1986.
    - A young mother bird struggles to provide food and security for her newly hatched baby. After some hardships, the mother bird finds she cannot adequately care for her young one. She makes the difficult decision to let two birds who can provide a stable home adopt her baby bird. IL: Ages 5-10

120. Bulla, Clyde. *Open the Door and See All the People.* New York: Crowell, 1972.

  - Sisters Jo Ann and Teeny and their widowed mother move to a city after a fire destroys their farm. The girls miss their mother, who goes to work, but they also long for their dolls lost in the fire. Jo Ann and Teeny discover a toy-lending library, where they can borrow dolls and adopt them after proving they will care for them. IL: Ages 7-10

121. Burgess, Linda Cannon. *The Art of Adoption.* New York: Norton, 1981.

  - This text is written for the adoptee, birth parents, adoptive parents, and perspective adoptive parents. Examples address the many relevant factors concerning adoption, including the role of birth parents, genetic concerns, the feelings of children and adolescents, the social agency's role, and the issue of sealed records. IL: Adult

122. Caines, Jeanette. *Abby.* New York: Harper and Row, 1973.

  - Young Abby delights in her mother's retelling about her arrival in their home when she was less than one year old. Abby's main questions are answered naturally and gently. Her family is black and includes an older sibling who sometimes teases her. IL: Ages 3-8

123. Cassedy, Sylvia. *Behind the Attic Wall.* New York: Crowell, 1983.

  - Maggie is shuffled around from place to place and is finally settled with two great-aunts. She is treated poorly by the aunts and has trouble coping with her environment. Eventually, Maggie is placed in a loving family that meets her needs. IL: Ages 12-18

124. Cohen, Shari. *Coping with Being Adopted.* New York: Rosen, 1988.

  - The common problems associated with being adopted are discussed, and ways for coping with adoption are offered. There are sections on transracial and handicapped adoptees as well as other issues related to the complexity of the adoption process. IL: Ages 11-15

125. Drescher, Joan. *Your Family, My Family.* New York: Walker and Company, 1980.

   - Various family forms are described: a two-parent family where both parents work, an adopted child's family, a family where child custody is shared by parents, and a foster family. The strengths of family life such as having a sense of belonging, sharing with others, and cooperating are emphasized. IL: Ages 4-8

126. DuPrau, Jeanne. *Adoption: The Facts, Feelings, and Issues of a Double Heritage.* New York: Messner, 1981.

   - This book presents an overview of the emotional, ethical, and legal questions related to adoption. The book answers many of the complex questions related to the adoption process and includes a focused look at the controversy over birth-history disclosure. IL: Ages 12-17

127. First, Julia. *I Rebekah, Take You, the Lawrences.* New York: Watts, 1981.

   - After a series of short-term foster care placements, twelve-year-old Rebekah is adopted by a warm and welcoming childless couple. She has mixed feelings about leaving the orphanage, fantasies about her biological parents, and feels shame at being adopted. Rebekah yearns to love and be loved, which happens gradually when a brother is adopted into the family as well. IL: Ages 8-12

128. Fisher, Iris L. *Katie-Bo: An Adoption Story.* New York: Adama, 1987.

   - This book is about an adopted Korean child. The book presents the emotions of biological children, including generosity and hostility, toward an adopted child. IL: Ages 5-9

129. Freudberg, Judy, and Geiss, Tony. *Susan and Gordon Adopt a Baby.* New York: Random House/Children's Television Workshop, 1986.

- This book tells how Susan and Gordon become parents of Miles by adopting him. The story emphasizes that now they will be Miles's parents forever, and that when someone new enters the family, the love just grows and grows. IL: Ages 3-7

130. Girard, Linda Walvoord. *Adoption Is for Always.* Niles, IL: Whitman, 1986.

- A small girl realizes she has been adopted and reacts with anger. She goes through various stages including grief, pain, loneliness, fear, curiosity about her biological parents, self-doubt, and finally, acceptance. Her adoptive parents give her support, love, and understanding. They assure her that they will always be her parents. IL: Ages 4-8

131. Gordon, Shirley. *The Boy Who Wanted a Family.* New York: Harper and Row, 1980.

- After years of being in a number of foster placements, seven-year-old Michael is about to be adopted. The proceedings take a full year, during which Michael feels tense about his adoption by a single woman. However, Michael adjusts well to his adoptive home. IL: Ages 6-9

132. Greenberg, Judith E., and Carey, Helen H. *Adopted.* New York: Watts, 1987.

- Sarah and Ryan are adopted siblings. The children also have friends who are adopted. The book includes photos of the children. IL: Ages 5-9

133. Hyde, Margaret O. *Foster Care and Adoption.* New York: Watts, 1982.

- This book describes trends in adoption and foster care. The author also discusses hard-to-place children, black market adoption, surrogate mothering, and the search for biological parents by adoptees. A number of case studies are presented. IL: Ages 13-18

134. Koehler, Phoebe. *The Day We Met You.* New York: Bradbury Press, 1990.

- This is a story about parents who adopt a young child. A mother and father talk about their joy and the excitement of preparing for the arrival of an adopted child. IL: Ages 2-5

135. Korschunow, Irina. *The Foundling Fox.* New York: Harper and Row, 1982.

- This is a story about a fox whose mother is killed by hunters. The fox is adopted by a vixen and her family. IL: Ages 5-8

136. Krementz, Jill. *How It Feels to Be Adopted.* New York: Alfred A. Knopf, 1982.

- Nineteen adopted children between the ages of eight and sixteen tell their stories and share their feelings. The children represent many adoptive situations; they are from varied ethnic backgrounds; some were adopted by single parents; some have handicapped siblings; and a few of the older children are involved in searches for their biological parents. All stress the special aspects of adoption. IL: Ages 8-18

137. Lapsley, Susan. *I Am Adopted.* New York: Bradbury Press, 1975.

- Charles is a happy child who knows he is adopted. He is a secure and busy preschooler. Charles knows that adoption means he will have a permanent family. IL: Ages 2-5

138. Lindsay, Jeanne Warren. *Pregnant Too Soon: Adoption Is an Option.* Buena Park, CA: Morning Glory, 1988.

- This book is for pregnant teenagers who must make decisions concerning their pregnancies. Adoption is presented as an alternative for the teenage parent. IL: Ages 13-18

139. Livingston, Carole. *Why Was I Adopted?* Seacaucus, NJ: Lyle Stuart, 1978.

- A variety of issues are addressed here, including reasons biological parents give up their children, how an adoption happens, and why. The fact that the adopted child is a unique and special person is stressed. IL: Ages 6-10

140. Mayhar, Ardath. *Carrots and Miggle.* New York: Atheneum, 1986.

- An orphaned child moves in with relatives. The child has difficulty adjusting to a new family. Even though the child has an opportunity to move to a different new family, she decides to stay with her present one. IL: Ages 10-18

141. McHugh, Elisabeth. *Karen's Sister.* New York: Morrow, 1983.

- Karen reacts to her newly adopted Korean sister and to the news of her mother's engagement to a man with three children. IL: Ages 11-13

142. McHugh, Elisabeth. *Karen and Vicki.* New York: Greenwillow, 1984.

- Karen and her sister Meghan, both adopted Korean children, must adjust to their mother's marriage to a man with three children. The adjustment does not come easy for the family. IL: Ages 10-12

143. Meredith, Judith. *And Now We Are a Family.* Boston: Beacon Press, 1971.

- How babies are adopted, why parents adopt, and why biological parents must sometimes place their children in adoption are explained. Complex issues such as illegitimacy are discussed, and a text is included for adults. IL: Ages 8-18

144. Miles, Miska. *Aaron's Door.* Boston: Little, Brown, and Company, 1977.

- After being deserted by their biological parents, Aaron and his younger sister are sent to an adoptive home. Aaron locks a door against the world, angry and envious of his younger sister's acceptance of their new adoptive home. Gradually, the gentle but powerful love of his adoptive parents shatters Aaron's self-imposed isolation. IL: Ages 5-9

145. Mills, Claudia. *Boardwalk with Hotel.* New York: Macmillan, 1985.

- Jessica finds out that she was adopted because her parents thought they could not have children. After she is adopted, her parents have biological children. Jessica feels she is second-best to her siblings and is convinced that she is loved less than they are by her adoptive parents. She gradually comes to terms with her feelings about her adoptive family. IL: Ages 9-12

146. Nickman, Steven. *The Adoption Experience: Stories and Commentaries.* New York: Messner, 1985.

 • A child psychiatrist who treats adoptive children presents commentaries on adoption. Included are stories about children in foster care and adoption, including the problems they face. Seven different stories on adoption are presented. IL: Ages 11-18

147. Pursell, Margaret. *A Look at Adoption.* Minneapolis: Lerner, 1977.

 • Questions frequently asked by children about adoption are answered. Photographs concerning adoption are included. IL: Ages 8-18

148. Rosenberg, Maxine B. *Being Adopted.* New York: Lothrop, 1984.

 • This book emphasizes the unique problems found in transracial and transcultural adoptions. Included are a seven-year-old of multiracial parents, a ten-year-old East Indian, and an eight-year-old Korean. IL: Ages 7-11

149. Scott, Elaine. *Adoption.* New York: Watts, 1980.

 • This look at the adoption process explains the role of the court and social services. An analysis of the influence of the biological parents and adoptive parents on the child's personality is overviewed. IL: Ages 10-12

150. Sobol, Harriet Langsam. *We Don't Look Like Mom and Dad.* New York: Coward, 1984.

 • A photo-essay on the lives of an American couple and their two Korean sons. The concerns of the children regarding their biological parents and ethnic heritage are presented. The family unit is depicted as having love, respect, and pride. IL: Ages 5-10

151. Tax, Meredith. *Families*. Boston: Little, Brown, and Company, 1981.

- Six-year-old Angie describes her own family, which includes a stepparent. She also tells about the family forms of various children she knows: a two-parent family, an adoptive family, and a single-parent family, as well as other family forms. Angie claims the important thing in all families is for members to love each other. IL: Ages 4-8

Foster Care

152. Adler, Carole. *The Cat That Was Left Behind.* New York: Clarion, 1981.

- Chad Lester, a thirteen-year-old foster child, has been sent to another foster home. A parallel is drawn between Chad and a stray cat. As Chad tames the cat and cares for it, he gradually comes to terms with the facts he has long denied–that his unmarried mother who now has married does not want him back with her. IL: Ages 10-14

153. Adler, Carole. *The Magic of the Glits*. New York: Macmillan, 1979.

- Two children of misfortune, thrown together for the summer, must make the best of it. Jeremy, a twelve-year-old, is recuperating from a broken leg. Lynette, a seven-year-old foster child, is placed in Jeremy's home. Problems begin to arise between Jeremy and Lynette; however, they are able to resolve them. IL: Ages 9-13

154. Anderson, Deborah, and Finne, Martha. *Jason's Story.* Minneapolis: Dillion Press, 1986.

- Seven-year-old Jason lives with his biological mother. For part of his life, Jason lived with foster parents. He was placed in foster care because his mother neglected him. The story of Jason helps foster children understand why they have been placed in care and learn to deal with the emotional conflicts related to placement. IL: Ages 5-10

155. Bunting, Eve. *If I Asked You, Would You Stay?* New York: Lippincott, 1984.

   - Crow has been rejected by his mother and placed in a series of foster homes. He runs away from his last foster home, not because he did not receive love and support but because he was afraid of another rejection. When Crow meets another child who has been abused, their relationship helps both children to adjust to problems they must face. IL: Ages 12-18

156. Byars, Betsy. *The Pinballs.* New York: Harper and Row, 1977.

   - Fifteen-year-old Carlie, thirteen-year-old Harvey, and eight-year-old Thomas have all been abused or neglected. The three children are placed with the Mason family. The children's reactions to placement include hostility, withdrawal, and depression. In time, the children feel more secure in the Mason's family. IL: Ages 11-18

157. Eige, Lillian. *Cady.* New York: Harper, 1987.

   - Cady runs away from his abusive aunt. He stays a while with a cousin, but one day he is told to leave. He moves from home to home. Cady is a classic example of how foster children feel—not feeling at home or safe with anyone. It is not clear what becomes of Cady's life. IL: Ages 9-12

158. Greenfield, Eloise. *Grandmama's Joy.* New York: Putnam, 1980.

   - In infancy, Rhondy is orphaned when her parents are killed. Rhondy is placed with her grandmother, who helps her deal with the pain of losing her biological parents. IL: Ages 14-18

159. Hahn, Mary Downing. *Daphne's Book.* New York: Clarion, 1983.

   - Daphne and her sister, Hope, live with their grandmother. Their parents have died, and their grandmother is emotionally troubled. Daphne and Hope are placed in an institutional setting; they eventually are placed with a cousin. IL: Ages 10-18

160. Hall, Lynn. *Mrs. Portree's Pony.* New York: Scribner's, 1986.

- It has been seven years since Addie's mother, Gloria, prevailed on her old friend, Alice, to take in her daughter because she did not want Addie living with them anymore. Alice cannot care for her anymore, and Addie is placed in loving foster care. Addie adjusts well to her new foster home and finally forgives her mother for not caring for her. IL: Ages 9-12

161. Holz, Loretta. *Foster Child.* New York: Messner, 1984.

- In this book, Peter tells his own story. His mother, abandoned by her husband, Peter's father, begins drinking heavily. No longer able to function as a parent, Peter's mother must place him in foster care. IL: Ages 9-12

162. Hyde, Margaret O. *Foster Care and Adoption.* New York: Watts, 1982.

- This book describes trends in adoption and foster care and discusses hard-to-place children, black market adoption, surrogate mothering, and the search for biological parents by adoptees. A number of case studies are presented. IL: Ages 13-18

163. MacLachlan, Patricia. *Mama One, Mama Two.* New York: Harper and Row, 1982.

- Mama One is Maudie's biological mother; Mama Two is Maudie's foster mother. Maudie is placed in foster care due to the emotional problems of her mother. Although Maudie was very depressed after placement, she begins to feel secure in her foster home and hopes to return to her biological mother. IL: Ages 4-8

164. McCutcheon, Elsie. *Storm Bird.* New York: Farrar, 1987.

- Jenny's father must go to sea, so he leaves her with an aunt. Jenny's mother is dead, and Jenny has a close, loving relationship with her father. Jenny experiences the loss of and separation from her father throughout the story. IL: Ages 13-18

165. Mebs, Gudrun. *Sunday's Child.* New York: Dial Books, 1986.

    • Ten-year-old Jenny finally is placed in a foster home after living in an orphanage as long as she can remember. IL: Ages 7-11

166. Myers, Walter Dean. *Won't Know Till I Get There.* New York: Viking, 1982.

    • Fourteen-year-old Stephen, a middle-income child, matures one summer when his parents decide to foster a less fortunate child. Earl, who has experienced numerous foster placements, is suspicious when he is placed with Stephen's family. The problems of both Stephen and thirteen-year-old Earl are described, including the difficulty of placing Earl for adoption. IL: Ages 11-15

167. Paterson, Katherine. *The Great Gilly Hopkins.* New York: Thomas Y. Crowell, 1978.

    • Abandoned by her mother eight years ago, eleven-year-old Gilly sets out to create trouble in her third foster home. Gilly mistreats another younger foster child and is extremely rude to her new foster parent, who is the first adult ever to really care about Gilly. When Gilly makes contact with her biological mother, she runs away to her but finds her mother doesn't really want her. Although Gilly finally forms an attachment to her foster mother, she must reluctantly leave to live with her grandmother. IL: Ages 10-14

168. Piepgras, Ruth. *My Name Is Mike Trumsky.* Chicago: Child's World, 1979.

    • Depicting the confusion foster children feel, this book shows that it is all right to love both foster parents and biological parents. The material on foster care is factual. IL: Ages 6-10

169. Wolitzer, Hilma. *Toby Lived Here.* New York: Farrar, Strauss, and Giroux, 1978.

    • Toby, a twelve-year-old, is placed in foster care with her younger sister, Anne. Toby feels insecure in the foster home, while Anne feels happy and secure. Eventually the girls' mother is able to care for her daughters again. Toby gradually adjusts to her foster home and even feels sad when she must return to her biological mother. IL: Ages 11-14.

170. Wosmek, Frances. *A Brown Bird Singing*. New York: Lothrop, 1985.

- Anego is a Native American. She lives with Anglo parents who provide emotional support to her. When she is treated poorly by Anglo children, this affects her self-esteem. Her biological father returns, and she is given the choice of leaving with her father or staying in her foster home. The reader is not informed of her choice. IL: Ages 9-12

SELF-DEVELOPMENT

171. Auw, Andrew. *Gentle Roads to Survival*. Boulder Creek, CO: Asian, 1991.

- The author offers a humanistic approach to self-development. A guide to making self-healing choices is offered. The book focuses on a number of areas that are critical to self-development including religion, morality, parenting, marriage, and crosscultural adaptation. IL: Adult

172. Bach, George, and Wyden, Peter. *How to Fight Fair in Love and Marriage*. New York: Avon Books, 1968.

- This book is about fair fighting in love and marriage. The work is based on the lead author's theory of constructive aggression. This theory suggests that conflict and fighting in close relationships are inevitable. The work concludes that what ails most marriages is a couple's inability to fight. When couples do not fight, they play games, get bored, and have misunderstandings and extramarital affairs. The work offers fighting tactics. IL: Adult

173. Basch, Michael Franz. *Understanding Psychotherapy: The Science Behind the Act*. New York: Basic Books, 1990.

- The author, a psychiatrist, explains how and why psychotherapy works. The book is written for those who are currently undergoing, or considering, treatment. IL: Adult

174. Bernard, Michael. *Staying Rational in an Irrational World.* New York: Carol Publishing, 1991.

 - This book applies cognitive therapy techniques to solving personal problems. The work offers the applications of rational emotive therapy as the core cognitive approach to problem solving in a number of areas including love, dating, sex, work, children, parents, women's issues, homosexuality, and death and dying. The basic theme of rational emotive therapy is that coping can be effectively accomplished by replacing irrational thinking with rational thinking. The book includes a number of examples in which individuals learn to talk to themselves more effectively and think in more rational ways. IL: Adult

175. Bly, Robert. *Iron John: A Book About Men.* Reading, MA: Addison-Wesley, 1990.

 - By retelling the Grimm Brothers' tale, the author explores the pain and confusion among contemporary men and points the way toward discovering a long tradition of male's approaches to feeling. IL: Adult

176. Bolles, Richard Nelson. *The 1992 What Color Is Your Parachute?* Berkeley, CA: Ten Speed Press, 1992.

 - This work is designed to help people change their lives. The book is written specifically for job-hunters and those who wish to change careers. IL: Adult

177. Caplan, Paula. *Don't Blame Mother: Mending in the Mother-Daughter Relationship.* New York: Harper and Row, 1989.

 - The theme of this book is that society and psychology have shortchanged mothers by too often blaming them for the shortcomings of their children. Daughters in particular are taught to criticize the work of mothering and to make their mothers the scapegoats for most problems they encounter in adulthood. The author underscores the value of women sharing experiences with each other as a means of personal change and self-improvement. Strategies for accomplishing this process are offered. IL: Adult

178. Cherry, Kittredge. *Hide and Seek.* San Francisco: Harper San Francisco, 1991.

- This book covers the problems associated with keeping or telling secrets about ourselves and others. A major focus of the work concerns the problems facing lesbians and gays who wish to come out. Advice is offered to lesbians and gays about this process. Self-discovery exercises are included. IL: Adult

179. Covey, Steven. *The 7 Habits of Highly Effective People.* New York: Simon and Schuster, 1989.

- This book offers approaches for readers on how to harness their potential to achieve their goals. The author suggests that self-improvement can occur in individuals if they do an in-depth examination of their perspectives on life and their value systems. The seven basic habits of effective people are as follows: (1) be proactive instead of reactive; (2) begin with the end in mind; (3) put first things first; (4) think win/win; (5) seek first to understand, then to be understood; (6) synergize; and (7) sharpen the saw (renewal). IL: Adult

180. Csikszentmihalyi, Mihaly. *Flow: The Psychology of Optimal Experience.* New York: Harper and Row, 1990.

- This work is about the optimal experiencing of life. Flow is the state of deep enjoyment and happiness that people feel when they have a sense of mastering life. Flow is a state of concentration in which a person becomes absorbed while engaging in activities. The work argues that flow can and should be controlled and not left to chance. The reader will discover that flow is the antidote to the twin evils of boredom and anxiety. Individuals can develop flow by setting challenges for themselves, by stretching themselves to the limit to achieve something worthwhile, by developing competent coping skills, and by combining the experiences of life into a meaningful pattern. IL: Adult

181. Cudney, Milton, and Hardy, Robert. *Self-Defeating Behaviors.* San Francisco: Harper, 1991.

- This is a cognitive and behavioral approach for eliminating a wide range of self-defeating behaviors. The author feels that we develop self-defeating behavior patterns such as defensiveness, procrastination, alcohol and drug abuse because they provide us with comfort and protection. These behaviors are obviously not the healthiest means of coping, and ultimately become problems because they become entrenched in our behavior patterns. A series of strategies are presented for freeing ourselves from self-destructive patterns of behavior. These include such activities as identifying the problem-causing behavior; specifying when, where, and with whom the behavior comes into play; intercepting the behavior while it is being practiced; and developing replacement techniques. IL: Adult

182. Dayton, Tian. *Drama Games: Techniques for Self-Development.* Deerfield Beach, FL: Health Communications, Inc., 1989.

    - Feelings are often attached to roles, according to this author. Thus, when we experiment with different roles, we naturally become more aware of a variety of feelings, by both expressing and experiencing them. This work helps individuals get in touch with and express hidden feelings in a safe and structured way, and offers ways in which individuals can be creative and spontaneous. IL: Adult

183. Dyer, Wayne W. *Pulling Your Own Strings: Dynamic Techniques for Dealing with Other People and Living Life as You Choose.* New York: HarperCollins Publishers, Inc., 1991.

    - The author offers a direct and practical guide for dealing with other people. The work also offers strategies for living life as one chooses. The author urges readers to be courageous and to realize what they can or cannot change about their lives. A number of self tests are included that help the readers monitor progress in learning how to take control of their live. IL: Adult

184. Dyer, Wayne W. *Your Erroneous Zones: Step by Step Advice for Escaping the Negative Thinking and Taking Control of Your Life.* New York: HarperCollins Publishers, Inc., 1991.

- The author provides step-by-step advice for escaping the trap of negative thinking. The work is designed to open the reader's mind and to improve social relationships with others. Strategies are offered for self-improvement and resolving personal issues. IL: Adult

185. Ellis, Albert, and Becker, Irving. *A Guide to Personal Happiness.* North Hollywood, CA: Wilshire Book Company, 1982.

- The authors suggest that individuals must search for personal happiness; no one else is going to do it for us. They argue that each of us has a right to personal happiness but that we need to seek it, even if it means putting ourselves first. The book includes Ellis's rational emotive techniques. IL: Adult

186. Ellis, Albert, and Harper, Robert. *A New Guide to Rational Living.* Englewood Cliffs, NJ: Prentice-Hall, 1975.

- This work offers a cognitive approach to self-fulfillment and happiness. The lead author of this work, Albert Ellis, developed rational emotive therapy and has written extensively on this approach to treatment. Rational emotive therapy concludes that people develop psychological problems because they use irrational beliefs to interpret what happens to themselves and their world. People disturb themselves by thinking in self-defeating, illogical, and unrealistic ways. In rational emotive therapy, the therapist takes an active role in interpreting the client's flawed thought processes, and suggests more rational approaches to dealing with problems. The book illustrates numerous cases between irrational thinkers and therapists and the subsequent interchanges that led to successful living. IL: Adult

187. Ellis, Albert, and Knaus, William. *Overcoming Procrastination: How to Think and Act Rationally in Spite of Life's Hassles.* New York: Institute for Rational Living, 1977.

- The work presents the cognitive therapeutic approach to rational emotive thinking in terms of performing life's tasks in a timely fashion. The authors define what procrastination means and its causes—low frustration tolerance, self-downing, and hostility. Rational emotive therapy is seen as the approach that can effectively help individuals overcome procrastination. IL: Adult

188. Fensterheim, Herbert. *Making Life Right When It Feels All Wrong*. New York: Rawlins Associates, 1988.

- The focus of this work is a modified behavioral approach to self-improvement. The author concludes that long-standing problems can be changed through a cognitive behavioral approach to self-improvement. The book applies this therapeutic approach to many different areas of life including assertiveness, work, love, friendships, and sports. Case studies are offered to illustrate the cognitive behavioral approach to self-improvement. IL: Adult

189. Fincham, Frank; Fernandes, Leyan; and Humphreys, Keith. *Communication in Relationships: A Guide for Couples and Professionals*. Champaign, IL: Research Press, 1993.

- This book applies knowledge from research and clinical practice to enhance relationships through improved communication. It is designed for people in a variety of situations, such as beginning, currently in, or thinking about ending a close relationship—or those working with others who are trying to improve their relationships. The book is also designed for people in different types of relationships including romantic, marital, multicultural, and gay or lesbian. IL: Adult

190. Forward, Susan. *Obsessive Love*. New York: Bantam, 1991.

- This book analyzes the type of destructive relationship in which passion holds a person prisoner. The work is designed for those who are obsessive lovers or their targets. Obsessive love is not really love at all, but rather a relationship that is dysfunctional. Obsessive behavior can range from relatively harmless efforts, such as compulsive phoning, to life-threatening acts. The work is designed to provide insight into various kinds of destructive relationships and what to do about them. IL: Adult

191. Frank, Victor. *Man's Search for Meaning.* New York: Pocket Books, 1984.

- This work presents an existentialist approach to the pursuit of self-fulfillment. This process is accomplished through logotherapy, a therapy aimed at helping individuals find meaning in their lives. The author suggests that the three most distinct human qualities are spirituality, freedom, and responsibility. These three areas are developed in the book and are critical to helping individuals find meaning in their lives. IL: Adult

192. Freeman, Arthur, and DeWolf, Rose. *The 10 Dumbest Mistakes Smart People Make and How to Avoid Them: Using Cognitive Therapy to Gain Greater Control of Your Life.* New York: HarperCollins Publishers, Inc., 1992.

- Cognitive therapeutic techniques are presented in this book. The focus is on the common habits of thinking that cause social maladjustment. These include the Chicken Little syndrome, perfectionism, comparisonism, and what-if thinking. A quiz is included that directs the reader to the appropriate chapter for solving a problem area. Techniques are recommended for changing one's thinking and behavior. IL: Adult

193. Fromm, Erich. *The Art of Loving.* New York: Harper and Row, 1956.

- This work is a philosophical and psychological treatise on the nature of love. Love is viewed as an attitude that determines one's relationship to the entire world. Love is an act of faith, a complete giving of oneself. Love, according to the author, involves a long and difficult learning process. This process requires discipline, concentration, patience, sensitivity to one's self, and the productive use of one's self. The author suggests that society greatly benefits when people learn to love. IL: Adult

194. Gergen, Kenneth J. *The Saturated Self: Dilemmas of Identity in Contemporary Life.* New York: Basic Books, 1992.

 - This is an analysis of how the realities of postmodern life are changing the way we view ourselves and our relationships. A goal of the work is to explain the contradictions of modern life. IL: Adult

195. Glasser, William. *Positive Addiction.* New York: Harper Perennial, 1976.

 - A psychological-based approach to positive thinking. The author argues that every person can overcome self-imposed weaknesses by engaging in positive addictions such as running and mediation. Negative addictions are escapes from the pain of striving for things people want but feel they cannot accomplish. Negative addictions include drinking, gambling, overeating, and smoking. Techniques for substituting positive addictions for negative addictions are offered. IL: Adult

196. Goldstein, Ross, and Landau, Diane. *Forty-Something: Claiming the Power and Passion of Your Midlife Years.* Los Angeles: Jeremy P. Tarcher, Inc., 1991.

 - The unique possibilities and advantages enjoyed by the seventy-six million baby boomers as they experience the midlife years are explored. The author offers ten skills for dealing with the midlife years. These include enhancing self-image. IL: Adult

197. Gotkin, Janet, and Gotkin, Paul. *Too Much Anger, Too Many Tears: A Personal Triumph Over Psychiatry.* New York: HarperCollins Publishers, Inc., 1992.

 - This work is a written account of one young woman's mental breakdown, years of psychiatric mistreatment, and eventual self-cure. The book is a statement against psychiatry. IL: Adult

198. Hagan, Kay Leigh. *Internal Affairs: A Journal Keeping Workbook for Self-Intimacy.* San Francisco: Harper San Francisco, 1990.

- Techniques are offered for journal keeping. The author illustrates how one can dig into one's past, and use this information to ultimately help one outline a personal map for the future. IL: Adult

199. Harris, Thomas. *I'm OK—You're OK.* New York: Harper and Row, 1967.

    - A classic in the field of self-help books. The work offers the transactional analysis approach to self-fulfillment. The author is a pioneer in the field of transactional analysis. Transactional analysis argues that people are responsible for their behavior in the present and future regardless of what has happened in the past. The author divides the personality into three parts: the Parent, the Adult, and the Child. The goal of transactional analysis is to strengthen and emancipate the Adult from the Parent and the Child. IL: Adult

200. Helmstetter, Shad. *What to Say When You Talk to Yourself.* Scottsdale, AZ: Grindle Press, 1986.

    - Provides advice on how to use self-talk to improve one's competence. The author offers behavioral techniques to complement the self-talk approach. The following self-talk techniques are presented: silent self-talk, self-speak, self-conversation, self-write, tape-talk, and creating self-talk tapes. The author offers self-talk approach as a useful strategy for changing attitudes, changing behaviors, and dealing with different situations. IL: Adult

201. Hendrix, Harville. *Getting the Love You Want.* New York: Henry Bolt, 1988.

    - A guide for couples who want to improve their relationships. The work offers numerous techniques for improving relationships based on awareness of unresolved childhood needs and conflicts that cause individuals to select particular spouses. Offered in the work is a ten-week course in marital therapy that teaches couples to communicate more clearly, to eliminate self-defeating behaviors, and to focus on meeting their partners' needs. IL: Adult

202. James, Muriel, and James, John. *Passion for Life: Psychology and the Human Spirit.* New York: Dutton, 1992.

   - This book offers seven basic spiritual urges that the authors feel shape human existence: (1) urge to live, (2) understanding, (3) creativity, (4) enjoyment, (5) connection, (6) transcending, and (7) freedom. The authors show that each of these are manifested in humans, and explain ways in which one can achieve them. IL: Adult

203. Jeffers, Susan. *Feel the Fear and Do It Anyway.* San Diego, CA: Harcourt Brace Jovanovich, 1987.

   - This book presents a cognitive approach to coping with fear. The author concludes that most people's inaction, whether it involves changing jobs, breaking off relationships, or starting new relationships, results from the fear of not being able to handle the consequence of these kinds of changes. The book describes fear as a sign that we are being challenged, and suggests that we should confront the fear by taking reasonable risks. IL: Adult

204. Johnson, Robert A. *Transformation: Understanding the Three Levels of Masculine Consciousness.* San Francisco: Harper San Francisco, 1991.

   - Using the literary archetypes of Don Quixote, Hamlet, and Faust, the author examines the three distinct levels of human consciousness development that each of these figures represents: The levels of consciousness explored are: the simple; the complex or three dimensional; and the redeemed or four dimensional. IL: Adult

205. Keen, Sam. *Fire in the Belly: On Being a Man.* New York: Bantam, 1991.

   - This book is written as a guide to the men's consciousness movement. The author looks at the stereotypes, myths, and evolving roles of contemporary men, and presents an alternative vision of virtue and virility for a modern age. New models of masculine spirit are offered, including what is wrong with men and women and their relationships. IL: Adult

206. Kopp, Sheldon. *Even a Stone Can Be a Teacher: Learning and Growing from the Experience of Everyday Life.* Los Angeles: Jeremy P. Tarcher, Inc., 1985.

- Events and activities of daily life experiences can be a source of growth and wisdom. The author illustrates how almost everything, from time spent watching soap operas to our reactions to illness and accidents, can be a source of profound inspiration and learning. IL: Adult

207. Kuenning, Delores. *Life After Vietnam: How Veterans and Their Loved Ones Can Heal the Psychological Wounds of War.* New York: Paragon House, 1991.

- This book is aimed at veterans who experience post-traumatic stress disorders. The effects of these disorders on relatives are also explored. The book offers advice for resolving guilt and grief for those affected by the Vietnam War experience. IL: Adult

208. Kushner, Harold. *When All You Ever Wanted Isn't Enough.* New York: Summit Books, 1986.

- The author offers a spiritually based approach to self-fulfillment based on his belief that material rewards create almost as many problems as they solve. This book suggests that there is not one big answer to life, but instead there are a series of answers. Answers are found in filling our day-to-day lives with meaning, with love of friends and family, and with striving for integrity. IL: Adult

209. Lakein, Alan. *How to Get Control of Your Time and Your Life.* New York: Signet, 1973.

- This book focuses on using time management to improve one's life. The author argues that time is life and that to be competent, individuals must manage time effectively. Advice is provided on how to find time we never knew we had, how to find to determine which tasks should be left undone, how to make the most of our priorities, how to create time for ourselves, when to slow down and when to speed up, the price paid when delaying, and finally, how to do better next time. IL: Adult

210. Miller, Joy. *My Holding You Back Up Is Holding Me Back: Recovery from Overresponsibility and Shame.* Deerfield Beach, FL: Health Communications, Inc., 1990.

   - This work explores the problem related to those who value others over their own selves. The consequences of over-responsibility can result in poor physical and emotional health. The author shows how to stop taking care of others and to start taking care of oneself. IL: Adult

211. Newman, Mildred, and Berkowitz, Bernard. *How to Be Your Best Friend.* New York: Random House, 1971.

   - This book presents ideas on how to like your self more and feel more self-fulfilled. The authors suggest that the road to self-fulfillment is to be more aware of one's accomplishments, to have compassion for ourselves, to praise our own achievements, and to be responsible for our choices. The format of the book is question and answer. IL: Adult

212. Peck, M. Scott. *The Road Less Traveled.* New York: Simon and Schuster, 1978.

   - This work offers psychological and spiritual approaches to self-fulfillment and happiness. The author concludes that life is difficult and, at times, a painful process. Strategies are offered that help clients deal with the problems of life. Four tools are offered to use as approaches to more successful living: delayed gratification, acceptance of responsibility, dedication to the truth, and balance. The work presents ideas for dealing with contemporary life. IL: Adult

213. Robbins, Anthony. *Unlimited Power.* New York: Fawcett Columbine, 1986.

   - A general approach to self-improvement is presented through the use of neurolinguistic programming. This theory argues that people can be programmed to be highly successful. A basic step to success, according to the author, is to select a successful person as a model and learn how that person became successful. Energy, passion, persistence of action, effective communication skills, and altruistic motives are all critical factors enhancing success and self-improvement. IL: Adult

214. Robinson, Bryan. *Stressed Out? A Guidebook for Taking Care of Yourself.* Deerfield Beach, FL: Health Communications, Inc., 1991.

   - This work is designed to help one evaluate one's stress quotient. The guidebook provides techniques on how to achieve a balanced, satisfying lifestyle. IL: Adult

215. Saltzman, Amy. *Downshifting: Reinventing Success on a Slower Track.* New York: HarperCollins Publishers, Inc., 1992.

   - The goal of this work is to show how one can achieve professional happiness on a slower track. The work is designed to help those who wish to make major changes in their lives. IL: Adult

216. Satir, Virginia. *Making Contact.* Berkeley, CA: Celestial Arts, 1976.

   - This work is aimed at helping individuals understand their full potential and improve interaction with others. Basic techniques are offered for making contact with others. IL: Adult

217. Satir, Virginia. *Meditations and Inspirations.* Berkeley, CA: Celestial Arts, 1985.

   - Based on the author's workshops, this work provides a series of meditations used by the author to help others enhance the self. IL: Adult

218. Satir, Virginia. *Self-Esteem.* Berkeley, CA: Celestial Arts, 1975.

   - The author focuses on the self-worth of the individual in modern society. The work is designed for those who are looking for new hope, new possibilities, and new positive feelings about themselves. IL: Adult

219. Satir, Virginia. *Your Many Faces.* Berkeley, CA: Cestial Arts, 1978.

- This book is designed to help the reader open doors and to make changes in one's life. The goal of the work is to help individuals make contact with the innermost self. IL: Adult

220. Scarf, Maggie. *Intimate Partners: Patterns in Love and Marriage.* New York: Random House, 1986.

- The author offers readers ways to solve their marital problems by understanding the stages that relationships go through and how our family of origin impacts marital relationships. The book is based on five married couples and analyzes their marital relationships in relation to the stages of the marriage cycle. These stages include: idealization, disenchantment, child rearing, career building, child launching, and the retirement years. IL: Adult

221. Schindler, John. *How to Live 365 Days a Year.* Englewood Cliffs, NJ: Prentice-Hall, 1975.

- This work presents an emotionally based approach to self-fulfillment. The author suggests that our illnesses and problems in life arise out of our emotions. The work is divided into two parts: Part I, How Your Emotions Make You Ill, suggests that emotions produce many physical diseases, and that there are good emotions and bad emotions. Part II, How to Cure Your Emotionally Induced Illness, describes how to attain emotional maturity within many areas of life including family, relationships, and at work. IL: Adult

222. Seligman, Martin. *Learned Optimism: The Skill to Conquer Life's Obstacle's Large and Small.* New York: Pocket Books, 1990.

- This book offers approaches for readers to learn to be optimistic about life. The author suggests that pessimism is learned, and can be unlearned. He concludes that there is a meaningful connection between positive thinking and health. IL: Adult

223. Simmermacher, Donald. *Self-Image Modification: Building Self-Esteem.* Deerfield Beach, FL: Health Communications, Inc., 1989.

• This book is designed for those who would like to develop a more positive self-image and self-esteem. Offered are systematic approaches aimed at actualizing human potential and growth. IL: Adult

224. Sternerg, Robert. *The Triangle of Love.* New York: Basic Books, 1987.

• The author discusses the different forms of love, which include sexual, romantic passion, the close emotional sharing of intimacy, and the enduring bond of commitment. The ultimate form of love includes all of these. Specific guidelines are offered for improving love relationships and the book includes a scale for measuring one's own love. IL: Adult

225. Stuart, Mary S., and Orr, Lynnzy. *Otherwise Perfect: People and Their Problems with Weight.* Deerfield Beach, FL: Health Communications, Inc., 1987.

• This book explores problems ranging from anorexia and obesity to codependency and its origins in the dysfunctional family. The authors provide a clear explanation of the complex varieties of eating disorders and how to cope with them successfully. IL: Adult

226. Taylor, Shelley. *Positive Illusions: Creative Self-Discipline and the Healthy Mind.* New York: Basic Books, 1989.

• This work is a psychologically based approach to positive thinking. The author stresses that when we face the complete truth about ourselves it is often a difficult task. It is argued that the healthy mind has a tendency to block out negative information; in turn, positive illusions help us cope. The work concludes that this creative deception is especially beneficial when we are threatened by adversity. IL: Adult

227. Walsh, Anthony. *The Science of Love: Understanding Love and Its Effects on Mind and Body.* Amherst, NY: Prometheus Books, 1991.

• The book offers an examination of the effects of love on one's physical and social well-being. The author covers the emotional, interactional, and physical aspects of love. IL: Adult

228. Ward, Joyce Rouser. *Therapy? Unmasking the Fears, Shattering the Myths, Finding the Path to Wellness.* Tarrytown, NY: Wynwood Press, 1992.

    - The author argues that self-help can only help so much when one cannot overcome self-destructive behaviors. Oftentimes seeking professional help is difficult because of the stigma attached to seeking such help. Steps are covered that help one decide on therapy, including how one should choose a therapist. The pain that emerges during therapy is also discussed. IL: Adult

229. Wegscheider-Cruse, Sharon. *Learning to Love Yourself: Finding Your Self-Worth.* Deerfield Beach, FL: Health Communications, Inc., 1987.

    - According to this text, self-worth is a choice, not a birthright. Approaches are offered to help one move from low self-esteem to the realization of one's own self-worth. The author concludes that one does not have to follow the family tradition of addiction or compulsion. IL: Adult

230. Weiss, Laurie. *I Don't Need Therapy but Where Do I Turn for Answers?* Deerfield Beach, FL: Health Communications, Inc., 1991.

    - This book provides answers to questions often asked by adult children recovering from emotional problems. The work includes problem-solving techniques. The author's goal is to help individuals get unstuck and move on with their lives. IL: Adult

231. Westin, Jeane Eddy. *The Thin Book.* Minneapolis: CompCare Publishers, 1989.

    - This work offers advice on losing weight. The author offers techniques that helped her lose weight. The work also presents information on self-understanding and self-awareness. IL: Adult

232. Wilson, Glenn D. *Your Personality and Potential: The Illustrated Guide to Self-Discovery.* New York: HarperCollins Publishers, Inc., 1992.

- This book examines the ways in which individual personalities develop, the advantages and problems inherent in the different personality types, the range of emotions experienced by all human beings, and what to do when emotional problems get out of hand. IL: Adult

SERIOUS ILLNESS

233. Arno, Peter S., and Feiden, Karyn. *Against the Odds: The Story of AIDS Drug Development, Politics, and Profits.* New York: HarperCollins Publishers, Inc., 1982.

- Information on the testing of drugs such AZT, ddl, Bactrin, gancyclovir, pentamindine, and Compound Q is offered. The role of government, pharmaceutical companies, activists, and patients, in the politics related to these drugs is presented. IL: Adult

234. Baur, Susan. *The Dinosaur Man: Tales of Madness and Enchantment from the Back Ward.* New York: HarperCollins Publishers, Inc., 1991.

- This book is based on the real-life experiences of those who have been hospitalized for schizophrenia. Many of the patients in the book are aware of their illness, while others often cannot distinguish between reality and illusion. The book provides insight into mental illness. IL: Adult

235. Bernstein, Richard K. *Diabetes: The Glucograf Method for Normalizing Blood Sugar.* Los Angeles: Jeremy P. Tarcher, Inc., 1989.

- This is a book designed to help diabetics self-monitor blood glucose levels. Information is provided on diet, nutrition, and exercise. IL: Adult

236. Broida, Helen. *Coping with Stroke: Communication Breakdown of Brain Injured Adults.* Austin, TX: Pro-Ed, 1979.

- Information and guidance are offered to victims of stroke. A question-and-answer format is utilized. The author responds to questions dealing with speech difficulties, writing, gestures, time, and changes that brain damage brings to families. IL: Adult

237. Budnick, Herbert N. *Heart to Heart: A Guide to the Psychological Aspects of Heart Disease.* New York: Health Press, 1991.

   - Heart disease can cripple the emotions as well as the body. This work shows how one can work effectively with individuals experiencing heart disease. The author illustrates the importance of the family in the treatment process. The work offers advice to heart disease victims and their families. IL: Adult

238. Callen, Michael. *Surviving AIDS.* New York: HarperCollins Publishers, Inc., 1991.

   - This is a chronicle of the struggle of long-term AIDS survivors. The book offers a message of help and inspiration for everyone affected by AIDS. IL: Adult

239. Carroll, David. *Living with Parkinson's.* New York: HarperCollins Publishers, Inc., 1992.

   - This is a guide for patients and caregivers based on the methods developed at a national center on aging. IL: Adult

240. Cooper, Peter. *Bulimia Nervosa and Binge-Eating: A Guide to Recovery.* New York: New York University Press, 1995.

   - Bulimia nervosa affects one in twenty women in the West. Concern about their shape and weight can drive women to such measures as prolonged fasting, excessive exercise, self-induced vomiting, and the taking of unnecessary laxatives in order to purge. This book takes a proactive approach, offering both a description of the disorder and a six-step plan for recovery. IL: Adult

241. Dreher, Henry. *Your Defense Against Cancer: The Complete Guide to Cancer Prevention.* New York: HarperCollins Publishers, Inc., 1990.

- This is a book designed for people who want to be healthy. The work is designed for the layperson. IL: Adult

242. Garrison, Judith G., and Shepherd, Scott. *Cancer and Hope: Charting a Survival Course.* Minneapolis: CompCare Publishers, 1989.

    - Written for those with cancer and their families and friends, this work is about taking control of one's life and participating in one's own healing. The author provides the metaphor of a sea journey to help the cancer patient. The work includes exercises, work sheets, visualizations, and thoughts to use to get well. IL: Adult

243. Gross, Amy, and Ito, Dee. *From Diagnosis to Recovery: Women Talk About Breast Surgery.* New York: HarperCollins Publishers, Inc., 1991.

    - This is a guide to the problems associated with breast surgery. Reactions to and feelings about breast surgery are presented. IL: Adult

244. Gross, Amy, and Ito, Dee. *Women Talk About Gynecological Surgery: From Diagnosis to Recovery.* New York: HarperCollins Publishers, Inc., 1992.

    - This guide for women describes all types of gynecological surgical procedures and tells the experiences of women who have been through them in their own words. A detailed glossary of terms and a section on patient's rights are presented. IL: Adult

245. Jampolsky, Gerald G. *Another Look at the Rainbows.* Berkeley, CA: Celestial Arts Publishing, 1983.

    - This work is written by and for children who have siblings afflicted with life-threatening illness. The drawings in the book are done by children, and demonstrate the pain, hurt, and fears they feel resulting from the knowledge that their siblings are seriously ill. IL: Adult

246. Klein, Allen. *The Healing Power of Humor.* Los Angeles: Jeremy P. Tarcher, Inc., 1988.

- This book is designed to help one turn negatives into positives. The author attempts to provide practical advice as to the fundamental importance of laughter and humor. IL: Adult

247. Krementz, Jill. *How It Feels to Live with a Physical Disability.* New York: S and S Trade, 1992.

- This is a series of life stories of children ranging in age from six to sixteen years. They share how it feels to live with a disability. The work is aimed at parents and professionals who work with children with disabilities. IL: Adult

248. The National Cancer Institute. *Chemotherapy and You.* Bethesda, MD: The National Cancer Institute, 1990.

- This book explains what chemotherapy is and how it works. The immediate and long-term effects of chemotherapy are explored. How to eat and drink during chemotherapy is discussed. The book also covers how chemotherapy and emotions interact, and how this interaction affects the patient, family, and friends. IL: Adult

249. The National Cancer Institute. *Help Yourself: Tips for Teenagers with Cancer.* Bethesda, MD: The National Cancer Institute, 1990.

- This work provides information and support to adolescents with cancer. Issues addressed include reactions to diagnosis, relationships with family and friends, school attendance, and body image. This book comes with an audiotape. IL: Adult

250. The National Cancer Institute. *Radiation Therapy and You.* Bethesda, MD: The National Cancer Institute, 1990.

- Practical ways to cope with the effects of radiation treatment are offered. These include the physical and emotional effects as well as the problems families and friends may encounter. The benefits and risks of radiation treatment, ways in which patients can cope with treatment, and the external and internal body changes that occur as a result of radiation therapy are discussed. IL: Adult

251. The National Cancer Institute. *Taking Time.* Bethesda, MD: The National Cancer Institute, 1990.

- This work discusses the issues cancer patients and their families face. This book helps cancer patients share their diagnosis with others and includes information on whom to tell and how to inform children and other significant people in the patient's life. It also focuses on helping patients share feelings with the family and in relating to the outside world. IL: Adult

252. The National Cancer Institute. *When Someone in Your Family Has Cancer.* Bethesda, MD: The National Cancer Institute, 1990.

- This book addresses young people whose parent or sibling has cancer. Includes information on cancer, its treatment, and emotional concerns. IL: Adult

253. Nelson, John E. *Healing the Split: A New Understanding of the Crisis and Treatment of the Mentally Ill.* Los Angeles: Jeremy P. Tarcher, Inc., 1991.

- Serious mental illness is the focus of this book. Drawing upon brain science, psychiatry, transpersonal psychology, and patient case histories, the author offers new strategies for dealing with serious mental illness. IL: Adult

254. Pantano, James A. *Living with Angina.* New York: HarperCollins Publishers, Inc., 1991.

- A cardiologist outlines the causes, effects, and treatment of angina. The author offers approaches for helping patient and doctor work together to deal with the problem of angina. IL: Adult

255. Shtasel, Philip. *Medical Tests and Diagnostic Procedures: A Patient's Guide to Just What the Doctor Ordered.* New York: HarperCollins Publishers, Inc., 1991.

- This is written for the layperson as a guide to understanding what to expect when a doctor orders one to have a diagnostic test or to visit a specialist. The goal of the book is to help patients be better-informed consumers. IL: Adult

256. Siegel, Bernie S. *Love, Medicine, and Miracles: Lessons Learned About Self-Healing from a Surgeon's Experience with Exceptional Patients.* New York: HarperCollins Publishers, Inc., 1988.

   • This book covers the process of self-healing and cases of remission of serious illness. Strategies are offered for patients coping with serious illness. IL: Adult

257. Siegel, Bernie S. *Peace, Love, and Healing: The Bodymind and the Path to Self-Healing—An Exploration.* New York: HarperCollins Publishers, Inc., 1990.

   • This work stresses the importance of learning how to talk to our inner selves, and give ourselves healing messages through meditation, visualization, and relaxation. The author explores the unity between the mind and body, and the path to self-healing with inspiring stories of patients and their remissions from serious illness. IL: Adult

258. Simonton, O. Carl; Matthews-Simonton, Stephanie; and Creighton, James. *Getting Well Again: A Step-by-Step Self-Help Guide to Overcoming Cancer for Patients and Their Families.* Los Angeles: Jeremy P. Tarcher, Inc., 1989.

   • This book examines how patients can deal with cancer. Psychological techniques are offered. IL: Adult

SUBSTANCE-RELATED DISORDERS

259. Ackerman, Robert J. *Growing in the Shadow: Children of Alcoholics.* Deerfield Beach, FL: Health Communications, Inc., 1986.

   • This work explores the world of children of alcoholics. The wisdom of twenty-one leading authorities in the field of children of alcoholics is included in this work. IL: Adult

260. Ackerman, Robert J., and Michaels, Judith A. *Recovery Resource Guide,* fourth edition. Deerfield Beach, FL: Health Communications, Inc., 1989.

- This work is designed for professionals and laypersons who need information on children of alcoholics, family and codependence, personal recovery, and helping agencies. The authors list over 1,000 resources that are available for recovery. IL: Adult

261. Al-Anon. *One Day at a Time in Al-Anon.* New York: Al-Anon Family Group Headquarters, 1973.
   - This book targets relatives and friends of alcoholics. The Al-Anon program, the focus of this work, uses the Twelve-Step recovery approach. Each day is viewed as a fresh opportunity for self-realization and growth through the Al-Anon approach. The work includes a daily message and reminder for the reader. IL: Adult

262. Alcoholics Anonymous World Services. *Alcoholics Anonymous: "The Big Book,"* third edition. New York: AA World Services, 1976.
   - This offers a step-by-step guide to recovery from alcoholism. These steps are aimed at achieving sobriety and serenity from the disease of alcoholism. IL: Adult

263. Andre, Pierre. *Drug Addiction: Learn About It Before Your Kids Do.* Deerfield Beach, FL: Health Communications, Inc., 1987.
   - This work focuses on cocaine. The problem of addiction and how it takes hold of its victims is explored. Topics included in the work cover intervention, hospitalization, and treatment follow-up. IL: Adult

264. Balis, Susan Adlin. *Beyond the Illusion: Choices for Children of Alcoholics.* Deerfield Beach, FL: Health Communications, Inc., 1989.
   - According to the author, children who grow up with an alcoholic parent exist in a world of illusion. An exploration of these illusions and their devastating impact on the individual is presented. Clinical details are offered, including analysis of strategies for change and how children of alcoholics can discover new choices that allow them to grow beyond the illusions created by parents. IL: Adult

265. Beattie, Melodie. *Beyond Codependency.* New York: Harper and Row, 1989.

   - The author describes the self-sabotaging behavioral patterns of codependency in which the codependent person over-cares for the addictive person. The book addresses healthy recovery, the role of recycling (falling into old bad habits) in recovery, and the role of positive affirmations. The work is based on a Twelve-Step program approach to recovery and Alcoholics Anonymous. IL: Adult

266. Black, Claudia. *It Will Never Happen to Me.* New York: Ballentine, 1981.

   - This book is designed to help children, adolescents, and adults cope with the problem of an alcoholic parent. The author describes the alcoholic cycle, and paints a vivid picture of the pitfalls alcoholics face. Also offered are various resources that can help relatives of alcoholics. IL: Adult

267. Bradshaw, John. *Healing the Shame That Binds You.* Deerfield Beach, FL: Health Communications, 1988.

   - The author argues that many people develop a range of problems, including addictions, codependencies, and compulsions, because of toxic shame. Toxic shame is present in individuals when they feel that things are hopeless and that they are worthless. The author feels toxic shame colors a person's entire sense of self. A person can end toxic shame through the process of externalizing it. This externalization process involves the liberation of the inner child, integrating disowned parts, loving the self, healing memories and improving self-images, confronting one's inner voices, coping with toxic shame relationships, and the awakening of the spiritual self. Therapeutic strategies are offered to accomplished the process of ridding the self of toxic shame. IL: Adult

268. Brady, Tom. *Sobriety Is a Learning Process.* Deerfield Beach, FL: Health Communications, Inc., 1985.

- A systematic program for learning to live a sober lifestyle is offered. The work is designed to be used by individuals and groups in the process of recovery. IL: Adult

269. Brown, Stephane; Beletis, Susan; and Cermak, Timmen. *Adult Children of Alcoholics in Treatment.* Deerfield Beach, FL: Health Communications, Inc., 1989.

- Working together at the Stanford Alcohol Clinic, these authors developed useful findings on the treatment of alcoholism. They argue that a more sophisticated approach needs to be taken in the development of knowledge related to alcoholism. IL: Adult

270. Childress, Alice. *A Hero Aren't Nothing but a Sandwich.* New York: Coward, McCann, and Geoghegan, 1973.

- A thirteen-year-old black heroin addict lives with his grandmother and stepfather. The child denies he has a problem and refuses treatment. Gradually he recognizes his problem and receives treatment. IL: Ages 11-18

271. Choices. *Choices.* Los Angeles: University of Southern California, 1987.

- The focus of this book is to help kids not to be hustled into drug abuse. The work offers eight lesson models in both Spanish and English. IL: Ages 6-10

272. Conrad, Barnaby. *Time Is All We Have.* New York: Dell, 1986.

- This work explores the author's treatment for alcoholism at the Betty Ford Center. The author focuses on the human side of alcoholism. IL: Adult

273. Dorris, Michael. *The Broken Cord.* New York: HarperCollins Publishers, Inc., 1989.

- This work reports on what it is like to parent a child with Fetal Alcohol Syndrome. An adoptive mother tells her personal story about what it is like to raise a Fetal Alcohol Syndrome child. IL: Adult

274. Fassel, Diane. *Working Ourselves to Death.* San Francisco: Harper San Francisco, 1992.

- This is an exploration of work addicts. The author explains how to distinguish between overwork and work addiction, and provides examples and case histories. Self-tests and charts guide the reader toward balance and serenity through various techniques, including inventories and daily work plans. IL: Adult

275. Fishman, Ross. *Alcohol and Alcoholism.* New York: Chelsea House, 1986.

- This book is for junior-high students needing solid material on the problem of alcohol use and alcoholism. IL: Age 12-15

276. Ford, Betty. *Betty: A Glad Awakening.* New York: Jove, 1988.

- Betty Ford, the former First Lady, shares her battle with chemical dependency. The author exposes a human side of alcoholism; also emphasized is the importance of helping others. IL: Adult

277. Gold, Mark S. *The Good News About Drugs and Alcohol: Curing, Treating, and Preventing Substance Abuse in the New Age of Biopsychiatry.* New York: Random House, 1991.

- Biopsychiatry applies the rigorous standards of science and medicine to the practice of psychiatry. The author illustrates how this approach can be used to fight alcohol and drug abuse. The work also covers prevention and education efforts that appear successful in combating chemical abuse in schools, the home, and the workplace. IL: Adult

278. Gordon, Barbara. *I'm Dancing As Fast As I Can.* New York: HarperCollins Publishers, Inc., 1989.

- A successful career as an award-winning television producer and a good relationship with a man she loved did not stop the author's world from falling apart when she was advised to discontinue use of Valium. This work focuses on that experience. IL: Adult

279. Greene, Sheppard. *The Boy Who Drank Too Much.* New York: Viking, 1979.

- A boy wrestles with his own drinking problem as well as his father's. Through treatment, the boy is able to deal with his drinking problem. IL: Ages 12-14

280. Hart, Stan. *Rehab: A Comprehensive Guide to the Best Drug-Alcohol Treatment Centers in the U.S.* New York: Harper-Collins Publishers, Inc., 1988.

    - This is an analysis of drug-alcohol treatment centers in the United States, aimed at both professionals and laypersons concerned with the problem of alcohol and chemical dependency. IL: Adult

281. Hawkes, Nigel. *The Heroin Trail.* Illustrated by Ron Hayward Associates. New York: Gloucestea Press, 1986.

    - This discussion of heroin pulls no punches. The text includes a pictorial presentation on heroin abuse. IL: Ages 11-14

282. Hewett, Paul. *Straight Talk About Drugs.* Minneapolis: Comp-Care Publishers, 1990.

    - This is a book that offers facts about drugs. The work is particularly designed for parents to give to young people. IL: Adult

283. Hyde, Margaret O., ed. *Mind Drugs.* New York: Dood, 1986.

    - This accurate presentation of drug abuse informs the reader about this serious problem. Counselors will find this text extremely helpful. IL: Age 12-18

284. Jampolsky, Lee. *Healing the Addictive Mind.* Berkeley: Cestial Arts, 1991.

    - This work offers approaches for freeing one's self from addictive patterns and relationships. The author suggests that the human conditions that affect most people, and create fixed in habits of thinking that keep one stuck, can be changed. The author offers strategies for bringing about these changes. IL: Adult

285. Kasi, Charlotte Davis. *Women, Sex and Addiction: A Search for Love and Power.* New York: HarperCollins Publishers, Inc., 1990.

- Sexual addiction and codependency are the focus of this work. The book provides a cultural analysis of the problem and offers solutions. IL: Adult

286. Kritsberg, Wayne. *Gifts: For Personal Growth and Recovery.* Deerfield Beach, FL: Health Communications, Inc., 1988.

    - Visualizations, affirmations, journal writing, and other techniques are offered as gifts for those who wish to recover from alcoholism. The work also stresses problems and issues related to codependency. IL: Adult

287. Marlin, Emily. *Relations in Recovery: New Rules, New Roles for Couples and Families.* New York: HarperCollins Publishers, Inc., 1990.

    - This work shows that it is possible to reestablish and restructure relationships that have floundered or failed under the burden of alcohol or other addictions. The significant changes in attitude and behavior that both codependents and the alcoholic or addict must make in order to break negative patterns are covered. The author emphasizes that the alcoholic or addict must heal old wounds, air resentments, and learn to deal with new ones as they arise. IL: Adult

288. May, Gerald C. *Addiction and Grace.* New York: HarperCollins Publishers, Inc., 1988.

    - This work offers spiritual and psychological principles to help combat any form of addiction. The author suggests that relationships with others are a major cause of all forms of addiction including drugs, sex, love, food, work, gambling, and so on. The book suggests that in order for one to recover from addiction, one must develop insight and the adoption of certain spiritual principles. IL: Adult

289. May, Gerald G. *The Awakened Heart: Living Beyond Addiction.* San Francisco: Harper San Francisco, 1991.

    - Love is viewed as an important component of one's social well-being. This book argues that the quest for efficiency and achievement distracts from people finding love. The author concludes that opening one's heart and trusting others will free one from addictive and compulsive behaviors. IL: Adult

290. Milam, James, and Ketcham, Katherine. *Under the Influence: A Guide to Myths and Realities of Alcoholism.* New York: Bantam, 1984.

   - This book is based on scientific research that examines the physical factors that set alcoholics and nonalcoholics apart. It offers a stigma-free way of understanding and treating alcoholism. IL: Adult

291. Mohn, Nicholas. *In Nueva York.* New York: Dial Press, 1977.

   - Rudi's diner is the hub of a poor ethnic neighborhood in New York City. Stories are told of many different people in the neighborhood with the diner serving as the place where their lives intersect. Alcohol and drugs are problems for several of the people. IL: Ages 14-18

292. Newman, Susan. *You Can Say No to a Drink or a Drug.* Photographs by George Tibboni. New York: Putnam/Perigee, 1986.

   - Through ten vignettes, this text shows kids ways of saying no to drugs and alcohol, even in the face of strong peer pressure. IL: Ages 10-14

293. O'Neill, Charles. *Focus on Alcohol.* Frederick, MD: Twenty-First Century Books, 1990.

   - This is a drug alert book designed to educate young people about the use and abuse of alcohol. Pressures to drink are examined from a number of different viewpoints. Could be adapted for group work with young people in middle school on such topics as self-esteem building. IL: Ages 10-14

294. Schaef, Anne Wilson, and Fassel, Diane. *The Addictive Organization.* San Francisco: Harper San Francisco, 1990.

   - The work focuses on the dysfunctional addictive systems in business and other organizations, specifically, how they operate, how to recognize them, and how to begin the, recovery process within them. IL: Adult

295. Seixas, Judith S., and Youcha, Geraldine. *Children of Alcoholism: A Survivor's Manual.* New York: HarperCollins Publishers, Inc., 1986.

    - Drawing on interviews with hundreds of adult survivors, the authors address the destructive patterns that can continue through a lifetime. They look at the shame and secrecy that typify the emotional makeup of a child of alcoholism, and discuss such feelings as guilt, embarrassment, and lack of self-esteem. IL: Adult

296. Shepherd, Scott. *Survival Handbook for the Newly Recovering.* Minneapolis: CompCare Publishers, 1988.

    - This book leads the newly recovering through the perils of the desert of low self-esteem, the swamp of boredom, the bitter wind of loneliness, and the mountains of depression. IL: Adult

297. Sikorsky, Ignor. *AA's Godparent: Three Early Influences on Alcoholics Anonymous.* Minneapolis: CompCare Publishers, 1990.

    - This work explores the influence of three nonalcoholics—psychiatrist Carl Jung, theologian Emmet Fox, and writer Jack Alexander—on Alcoholics Anonymous. It is designed for people who wish to know more about Alcoholics Anonymous. IL: Adult

298. Strasser, Todd. *Angel Dust Blues.* New York: Coward, McCann, and Geoghegan, 1979.

    - When a wealthy seventeen-year-old youngster becomes bored with life, he turns to the drug culture for excitement. IL: Ages 13-18

299. Thomsen, Robert. *Bill W.* New York: HarperCollins Publishers, Inc., 1985.

    - This work focuses on the genesis of Alcoholics Anonymous. Insight is offered into the mind of the founder of AA. IL: Adult

300. Whitfield, Charles L. *A Gift to Myself: A Personal Guide to Healing My Child Within.* Deerfield Beach, FL: Health Communications, Inc., 1990.

- This work provides deeper exploration into how to heal our child within. The goal of the work is to help one experience the gift of creating personal freedom in recovery and in one's life. IL: Adult

301. Whitfield, Charles L. *Healing the Child Within: Discovery and Recovery for Adult Children of Dysfunctional Families.* Deerfield Beach, FL: Health Communications, Inc., 1987.

- The audience for this work is those who are in the process of recovery from a troubled or dysfunctional family. The work explores the different forms of abuse, shame, lack of boundaries, codependence, and compulsion. The author offers approaches to recognize the symptoms of codependency and how to heal them. IL: Adult

302. Woititz, Janet G. *Adult Children of Alcoholics.* Deerfield Beach, FL: Health Communications, Inc., 1990.

- What children of alcoholics need is basic information to sort out the effects of alcoholism. The author provides this information. IL: Adult

Chapter 5

Bibliotherapy and Clinical Social Work

It has been known for a number of years that books can provide comfort and support to readers. Recently, the formalized use of books in treatment has evolved to what is now known as bibliotherapy. Bibliotherapy is a useful approach for helping individuals deal with psychological, social, and developmental problems. This work' illustrates how bibliotherapy can be used as a therapeutic tool. Useful strategies are presented for implementing bibliotherapy for complex psychological problems, as well as helping children and adults deal with basic developmental needs.

Bibliotherapy can be defined in a number of ways. The term bibliotherapy, most simply defined, means helping individuals through the use of books. In the clinical literature, the term bibliotherapy is also referred to as bibliocounseling, bibliopsychology, biblioeducation, biblioguidance, library therapeutics, biblioprophylaxis, tutorial group therapy, and literatherapy. Virtually everyone has used bibliotherapy to cope with issues and problems faced throughout the life cycle. For example, it has been the experience of the author that when an individual is faced with a serious problem, he or she will almost always ask if books are available on the problem. In fact, as noted in this work, psychologists, psychiatrists, and related professionals often prescribe books as a strategy for helping clients initially cope with problems (Starker, 1988). Social work practitioners' will find that books can help clients conduct self-examination and provide them with insight into countless types of problems, and that reading material can range from fiction to self-help books.

Regardless of the source of reading materials, Bernstein (1989) argues that certain salient factors must be present for bibliotherapy to occur. First, the author of a written work must communicate to a reader in either aesthetic form or through discourse; the reader, in turn, must understand and respond to the work before attitudinal and/or behavioral changes can occur. Changes in attitudes or behavior can be brought about with the help of the practitioner or simply be self-induced. According to Bernstein, adults and children are typically the prime seekers of their own help through books. Bernstein (1989) wrote the following:

> Both adults and children are often the prime seekers of their own help through books, delegating an adult to a lesser role as facilitator. Lest any person protest they have never sought out books to help themselves, let them think back to a time they hid a book. In some manner, that book probably helped them—by providing information they were afraid or ashamed to seek elsewhere, by clarifying concepts, by explaining a bit of their own lives. (p. 159)

Bernstein clearly conveys the idea in the above quote that we all have used bibliotherapy in some shape or form, and that books are a very important source of helping many to cope with problems of daily life.

BIBLIOTHERAPY AND CLINICAL INTERVENTION

Social work practitioners will find that fiction and self-help books can enhance clinical practice. Ellis (1995) suggests that many emotionally troubled people learn more by reading than by interacting with a therapist or group. Those who are "allergic" to bibliotherapy can do well with audio and video materials. Many clients can deepen their emotional improvement by using books as part of their treatment. However, unfortunately, some individuals object to the time and expense required for individual or group therapy and prefer to use books when they might better benefit from regular treatment.

Being in treatment is no longer considered to be as disgraceful as it once was; still, millions of individuals stay away from it because of their feelings of shame about participating in and about being identified as in therapy. Even though treatment is important for these kinds of individuals, Ellis (1995) suggests these avoiders benefit considerably from books focusing on problems that confront them. Thousands of people live in communities where few or no therapists are available and where they would have to travel long distances to engage in face-to-face sessions; books are easily available to them. For example, people who participate in self-help groups, such as Alcoholics Anonymous, often do a great deal of reading and tape listening to supplement the help they get from a group. A therapist may never be involved in this phase of the recovery process.

Practitioners in the field of social work must realize that the self-help movement is well entrenched in American society. The use of books as a therapeutic tool is a key ingredient of this movement. Even though it is clearly understood that individuals should seek professional help when confronted with critical life issues, many do not. Practitioners must learn to adapt their practices to this new environment. It is important to learn about not only the limitations of books as a self-help tool, but also their strengths. This work explores the importance of books as a self-help tool. It particularly emphasizes how practitioners can use books as an adjunct to clinical intervention.

MANAGED CARE AND SELF-HELP BOOKS

As many social work practitioners now realize, managed care is an emerging service delivery approach in the fields of medicine and mental health. The aim of managed care is to control costs, improve client access to treatment, and move clients from a passive to an active role in the treatment process.

As found in the managed care approach to medical treatment, managed mental health care means that treatment and intervention are carefully monitored by third party payers. In the field of mental health, this approach is supposed to result in the most efficient use of resources and the highest quality treatment possible to clients, while at the same time containing costs. Within the field of mental health, managed care generally emphasizes short-term treatment and measurable goals. For example, the length of allowable stay for a client in a substance abuse program is often short term; the treatment typically emphasizes raising levels of the client's social functioning with specific behavioral objectives through the utilization of a wide range of techniques (Popple and Leighninger, 1996).

Self-help books can be viewed as useful tools that compliment a managed care approach to mental health. Specifically, self-help books can provide didactic information to clients that has traditionally been obtained through psychotherapy. More important, self-help books allow a client to play an active role in the diagnosis and treatment process. This role empowers the client, and also contributes to containing costs. Self-help books not only promote collaboration between therapist and client; books can also be used as preventative tools in a variety of problem areas including drug and alcohol prevention (Pardeck, 1994).

Managed care is aimed at delivering efficient and cost-effective treatment in the fields of medicine and mental health. Self-help books compliment the managed care approach to intervention because both stress client empowerment and the active participation of the client in all phases of the treatment process. In fact, there are a number of self-help books available that call for minimal support from the therapist during the treatment process. The service delivery system in mental health care is changing due to managed care; these evolutionary changes are calling for greater participation of clients in the treatment process which self-help books can promote.

FICTION AND BIBLIOTHERAPY

When the social work practitioner decides to use fiction as part of the bibliotherapeutic process, the following points should be considered. As stressed earlier in this work, the problem the client is facing is the most important factor in selecting a fiction book for treatment. The client's interest level, reading level, and alternate forms of book publication must also be taken into account.

The practitioner should consider the client's interest and reading levels as well as the presenting problem in selecting a fiction book for therapy. Chronological age and the level of maturity of the client largely determine the client's interest level. A too-difficult book can hamper the bibliotherapeutic process; a book with a reading level much lower than the client's may prove insulting.

Another element of book selection is the form of publication. Many fiction books are available in paperback form, which is more appealing to young people. Certain books have been developed in the forms of braille, talking books, or large type for use with individuals with disabilities. It is also critical for the social work practitioner to read the fiction book prior to its use in treatment. This will help to ensure that the book offers a realistic presentation of a presenting problem and also helps the practitioner focus on book content that will facilitate the bibliotherapeutic process.

Finally, if the practitioner decides to use fiction, often times in the form of novels, the stages of the bibliotherapeutic process must occur. Specifically, the client must be able to identify with a book character. The practitioner in turn must be skilled at moving the client through the processes of *identification and projection, abreaction and catharsis,* and *insight and integration.* As suggested earlier, clinicians who have a psychodynamic orientation to practice prefer fiction books as an adjunct to treatment.

NONFICTION SELF-HELP BOOKS AND BIBLIOTHERAPY

A number of strategies have been offered for choosing nonfiction self-help books (Santrock, Minnett, and Campbell, 1994). The following points offer additional tips for identifying quality nonfiction self-help books. Many of these books offer clinical activities that will enhance clinical intervention.

Do Not Select a Book Based Solely on Its Cover

The self-help book business is a very large business. Publishers spend huge sums of money to create glitzy titles that suggest they offer a major breakthrough for treating a certain kind of clinical problem. Both good and bad self-help books are produced and promoted by publishers. The social work practitioner should be skeptical of anything that sounds too wondrous. Any self-help book that suggests it is a cure for every possible problem should be avoided.

Select Self-Help Books That Recognize Multiple Causes of Problems

Clinical problems have complex causes. Oftentimes people look for a simple answer to solve complex problems; self-help books that provide such answers should be avoided. Clinical problems often have biological, psychological, and social causes. Efforts should be made by the practitioner to find self-help books that enhance this orientation to practice.

Closely Examine the Evidence Supporting the Self-Help Book

Many self-help books are not based on reliable scientific or clinical evidence. Oftentimes the author of a self-help book simply provides a testimony about the book's effectiveness in treating a problem. Always be skeptical of the author's claims about a book's effectiveness. Take a close look at the methodology used to support the author's claims concerning the self-help book's effectiveness.

Review the Author's Professional Credentials

Many of the self-help books recommended in this work are written by trained professionals in the fields of psychiatry, psychology, and counseling. The professional credentials of the author should be clearly noted in the chosen book; if they are not, the social work practitioner should probably avoid using it. Always be skeptical of authors who attack the field of mental health. The work of these authors typically has questionable merit and may even do damage to individuals.

CONCLUSION

As emphasized earlier in this work, social work practitioners have not traditionally used bibliotherapy as part of their practice, although bibliotherapy is a well-established practice technique in other professions including psychiatry and psychology. The goal of this book is to offer an orientation to bibliotherapy that social work practitioners should find useful. Strategies for using this novel tool in social work practice are offered. Social workers will find that many of these strategies are highly effective with a variety of clinical problems. It is stressed that bibliotherapy can be conducted through both fiction and nonfiction self-help books.

Bibliotherapy in a certain sense has been a part of the human experience since the creation of books. Numerous mental health practitioners now realize that individuals often use books as an initial source for understanding a problem; this insight has lead to the acceptance of bibliotherapy as a helpful therapeutic tool that can enhance the assessment and treatment process. Social workers will find that books can be a powerful tool for changing the lives of people.

References

Chapter 1

Aldridge, J., and Clayton, G. (1990). Sources of self-esteem: Perceptions of education majors. *College Student Journal,* 24; 404-409.

Bailey, C. A. (1982). Effects of therapist contact and a self-help manual in the treatment of sleep-onset insomnia. *Dissertation Abstracts International.*

Barker, R. L. (1995). *The social work dictionary,* second edition. Silver Spring, MD: NASW.

Baruth, L., and Burggraf, M. (1984). The counselor and single-parent families. *Elementary School Guidance and Counseling,* 19; 30-37.

Bernstein, J. (1983). *Books to help children cope with separation and loss.* (Second edition). New York: Bowker Company.

Bernstein, J. (1989). Bibliotherapy: How books can help children cope. In M. Rudman (Ed.), *Children's literature: Resource for the classroom.* New York: Christopher Gordon Publishers, Inc.; 159-173.

Berry, I. (1978). Contemporary bibliotherapy: Systematizing the field. In E. J. Rubin (Ed.), *Bibliotherapy sourcebook.* Phoenix, AZ: Oryx Press; 185-190.

Black, D. R., and Threlfall, W. E. (1986). A stepped approach to weight control: A minimal intervention and a bibliotherapy problem-solving program. *Behavior Therapy,* 17; 144-157.

Black, M. J. (1981). The empirical evaluation of a self-administered conversational training program. *Dissertation Abstracts International,* 42, 1596B. (University Microfilms No. 85-23, 265)

Bohlmann, N. A. (1986). Use of RET bibliotherapy to increase self-acceptance and self-actualization levels of runners. *Dissertation Abstracts International,* 46, 2191A. (University Microfilms No. 85-23, 265)

Cohen, L. J. (1993). The therapeutic use of reading: A qualitative study. *Journal of Poetry Therapy,* 7; 73-83.

Coleman, M., and Ganong, L. H. (1990). The use of juvenile fiction and self-help books with stepfamilies. *Journal of Counseling and Development,* 68; 327-331.

Conner, C. N. (1981). The effectiveness of bibliotherapy on teaching initiator dating skills to females. *Dissertation Abstracts International,* 42, 3818B. (University Microfilms No. 82-03, 109)

Cuevas, J. L. (1984). Cognitive treatment of chronic tension headache. *Dissertation Abstracts International,* 46, 955B. (University Microfilms No. 85-10, 012)

DeFrances, J., Dexter, R., Leary, T. J., and MacMullen, J. R. (1982). The effect of bibliotherapy and videotaping techniques on collective and self-concept formation in behaviorally disordered youth. *Proceedings of the 60th Annual International Convention of the Council for Exceptional Children.* Houston, TX. (ERIC Document Reproduction Service No. ED 218 885)

Dodge, L. T., Glasgow, R. E., and O'Neill, H. K. (1982). Bibliotherapy in the treatment of female orgasmic dysfunction. *Journal of Consulting and Clinical Psychology,* 50; 442-443.

Doll, B., and Doll, C. (1997). *Bibliotherapy with young people: Librarians and mental health professionals working together.* Englewood, CO: Libraries Unlimited, Inc.

Ellis, A. (1993). The advantages and disadvantages of self-help therapy materials. *Professional Psychology, Research and Practice,* 24; 335-339.

Farkas, G. S. and Yorker, B. (1993). Case studies of bibliotherapy. *Issues in Mental Health Nursing,* 14; 337-347.

Ford, J. D., Bashford, M. B., and DeWitt, K. N. (1984). Three approaches to marital enrichment: Toward optimal matching of participants and interventions. *Journal of Sex and Marital Therapy,* 10; 41-48.

Forest, J. J. (1991). Effects of attitudes and interests on personality change induced by psychological self-help books. *Psychological Reports,* 68; 587-592.

Frankel, M. J., and Merbaum, M. (1982). Effects of therapist contact and a self-control manual on nailbiting reduction. *Behavior Therapy,* 13; 125-129.

Gaffney, D. (1993). Bibliotherapy for girls: Read two books and see me in the morning. *Academic Nurse,* 11; 6-9.

Galliford, J. E. (1982). Eliminating self-defeating behavior: The effects of ESDB bibliotherapy compared to ESDB group therapy on weight control in women. *Dissertation Abstracts International,* 43, 1978B (University Microfilms No. 82-84, 784)

Giblin, P. (1989). Use of reading assignments in clinical practice. *The American Journal of Family Therapy,* 17; 219-228.

Giles, L. P. (1986). Effects of reading-mediated vicarious reinforcement on the behavior of disturbed children. *Dissertation Abstracts International,* 47, 4299B. (University Microfilms No. 87-02, 267)

Gould, R. A., Clum, G. A., and Shapiro, D. (1995). The use of bibliotherapy in treatment of panic disorders: A preliminary investigation. *Behavior Therapy,* 24; 241-252.

Griffin, B. (1984). *Special needs bibliography: Current books for/about children and young adults.* DeWitt, NY: Griffin.

Halliday, G. (1991). Psychological self-help books: How dangerous are they. *Psychotherapy,* 28; 678-680.

Harbaugh, J. K. (1984). The effectiveness of bibliotherapy in teaching problem solving skills to female juvenile delinquents. *Dissertation Abstracts International,* 45, 3072A. (University Microfilms No. 84-29, 693)

Klingman, A. (1985). Responding to a bereaved classmate: Comparison of two strategies for death education in the classroom. *Death Studies,* 9; 449-454.

Lanza, M. L. (1996). Bibliotherapy and beyond. *Perspectives in Psychiatric Care,* 52; 12-14.

Lesser, I. M. (1991). The treatment of panic disorders: Pharmacologic aspects. *Psychiatric Annuals,* 21; 341-346.

Libman, E., Fichten, C. S., Brender, W., Burstein, R., Cohen, J., and Binik, Y. M. (1984). A comparison of three therapeutic formats in the treatment of secondary orgasmic dysfunction. *Journal of Sex and Marital Therapy,* 10; 147-159.

Long, N., Rickert, V., and Ashcraft, E. (1993). Bibliotherapy as an adjunct to stimulant medication in treatment of attention-deficit hyperactivity disorder. *Journal of Pediatric Health Care,* 7; 82-88.

Marx, J. A., Gyorky, Z. K., Royalty, G. M., and Stern, T. E. (1992). Use of self-help books in psychotherapy. *Professional Psychology, Research and Practice,* 23; 300-305.

Matthews, D., and Lonsdale, R. (1992). Children in hospitals: Reading therapy and children in hospitals. *Health Libraries Review,* 9; 14-26.

Menninger, K. A. (1945). *The human mind.* New York: A. A. Knopf.

Miller, D. L. (1982). Effect of a program of therapeutic discipline on the attitude, attendance, and insight of truant adolescents. *Dissertation Abstracts International,* 43, 1048A. (University Microfilms No. 82-20, 323)

Morris-Vann, A. M. (1983). The efficacy of bibliotherapy on the mental health of elementary students who have experienced a loss precipitated by parental unemployment, divorce, marital separation or death. *Dissertation Abstracts International,* 44, 676A. (University Microfilms No. 83-15, 616)

Ogles, B. M., Lambert, M. J., and Craig, D. E. (1991). Comparison of self-help books for coping with loss: Expectations and attributions. *Journal of Counseling Psychology,* 38; 387-395.

Orton, G. L. (1997). *Strategies for counseling with children and their parents.* Pacific Grove, CA: Brooks/Cole Publishing.

Pardeck, J. A., and Pardeck, J. T. (1984). *Young people with problems: A guide to bibliotherapy.* Westport, CT: Greenwood Press.

Pardeck, J. A., and Pardeck, J. T. (1986). *Books for early childhood: A developmental perspective.* Westport, CT: Greenwood Press.

Pardeck, J. T. (1991a). Bibliotherapy and clinical social work. *Journal of Independent Social Work,* 5; 53-63.

Pardeck, J. T. (1991b). Using books in clinical practice. *Psychotherapy in Private Practice,* 9; 105-119.

Pardeck, J. T. (1993). *Using bibliotherapy in clinical practice: A guide to self-help books.* Westport, CT: Greenwood Press.

Pardeck, J. T., and Markward, M. J. (1995). Bibliotherapy: Using books to help children deal with problems. *Early Child Development and Care,* 106; 75-90.

Pardeck, J. T., and Pardeck, J. A. (1983). Using bibliotherapy in clinical practice with children of separation and divorce. *Arete,* 8; 10-17.

Pardeck, J. T., and Pardeck, J. A. (1987). Using bibliotherapy to help children cope with the changing family. *Social Work in Education,* 9; 107-116.

Pardeck, J. T., and Pardeck, J. A. (1989). Bibliotherapy: A tool for helping preschool children deal with developmental change related to family relationships. *Early Child Development and Care,* 47; 107-129.

Pezzot-Pearce, T. D., LeBow, M. D., and Pearce, J. W. (1982). Increasing cost-effectiveness in obesity treatment through use of self-help behavioral manuals and decreased therapist contact. *Journal of Consulting and Clinical Psychology,* 50; 448-449.

Psychotherapy Newsletter. (1994). Using bibliotherapy responsibly. Providence, RI: Author.

Ray, R. D. (1983). The relationship of bibliotherapy, self-concept and reading readiness among kindergarten children. *Dissertation Abstracts International,* 45, 140A. (University Microfilms No. 84-02, 425)

Rosen, G. M. (1981). Guidelines for the review of do-it-yourself books. *Contemporary Psychology,* 26; 189-191.

Rosen, G. M. (1987). Self-help treatment books and the commercialization of psychotherapy. *American Psychologist,* 42; 46-51.

Rubin, R. (1978). *Using bibliotherapy: A guide to theory and practice.* Phoenix, AZ: Oryx Press.

Rucker, J. P. (1983). An outcome study of two short-term weight loss methods: Bibliotherapy and interpersonal growth group therapy. *Dissertation Abstracts International,* 44, 2421A.

Sadler, M. S. (1982). The effects of bibliotherapy on anomie and life satisfaction of the elderly. *Literature, Literary Response, and the Teaching of Literature.* Abstracts of doctoral dissertations published in *Dissertation Abstracts International, January through June 1983* (Vol. 43, Nos. 7-12). (ERIC Document Reproduction Service No. ED 230 983)

Santrock, J. W., Minnett, A. M., and Campbell, B. D. (1994). *The authoritative guide to self-help books.* New York: The Guilford Press.

Shafron, P. W. (1983). Relationship between bibliotherapy and the self-esteem of junior high school students enrolled in remedial reading classes. *Dissertation Abstracts International,* 44, 1037A. (University Microfilms No. 83-18, 314)

Shechtman, Z. (1994). Challenging teacher beliefs via counseling methods: A descriptive study. *Teaching Education,* 6; 29-40.

Shrodes, C. (1949). Bibliotherapy: A theoretical and clinical study. Doctoral Dissertation: University of California.

Standley, F., and Standley, N. (1970). An experimental use of black literature at a predominantly white university. *Research in Teaching English,* 4; 139-148.

Starker, S. (1986). Promises and prescriptions: Self-help books in mental health and medicine. *American Journal of Health Promotion,* 2; 19-24, 68.

Starker, S. (1988). Psychologists and self-help books: Attitudes and prescriptive practices of clinicians. *American Journal of Psychotherapy,* 42; 448-455.

Starker, S. (1992a). Self-help books: Ubiquitous agents of health care. *Medical Psychotherapy: An International Journal,* 3; 187-194.

Starker, S. (1992b). Characteristics of self-help book readers among VA medical outpatients. *Medical Psychotherapy: An International Journal,* 6; 89-93.
Starker, S. (1994). Self-care materials in the practice of cardiology: An explorative study among American cardiologists. *Patient Education and Counseling,* 24; 91-94.
Swantic, F. M. (1986). An investigation of the effectiveness of bibliotherapy on middle grade students who repeatedly display inappropriate behavior in the school setting. *Dissertation Abstracts International,* 47, 843A.
Tatara, W. (1964). Effects of novels on ideas about scientists. *Journal of Educational Research,* 58; 3-9.
Taylor, V. W. (1982). An investigation of the effect of bibliotherapy on the self-concepts of kindergarten children from one-parent families. *Dissertation Abstracts International,* 43, 3505A. (University Microfilms No. 83-06, 465)
Warner, R. E. (1991). Self-help book prescription practices of Canadian university counsellors. *Canadian Journal of Counseling,* 25; 359-362.
Webster's New Collegiate Dictionary. (1981). Springfield, MA: Merriam-Webster.
Wilson, J. (1951). The treatment of attitudinal pathosis by bibliotherapy: A case study. *Journal of Clinical Psychology,* 7; 345-351.
Zaccaria, J., and Moses, H. (1968). *Facilitating human development through reading: The use of bibliotherapy in teaching and counseling.* Champaign, IL: Stipes.

Chapter 2

Barker, R. L. (1995). *The social work dictionary,* second edition. Silver Springs, MD: NASW.
Bernstein, J. (1989). Bibliotherapy: How books can help children cope. In M. Rudman (Ed.), *Children's literature: Resource for the classroom.* New York: Christopher Gordon Publishers, Inc., 159-173.
Craighead, L., McNamara, K., and Horan, J. (1984). Perspectives on self-help and bibliotherapy: You are what you read. InS. Brown and R. Lent (Eds.) *Handbook of counseling psychotherapy.* New York: John Wiley and Sons, 878-929.
Doll, B., and Doll, C. (1997). *Bibliotherapy with young people: Librarians and mental health professionals working together.* Englewood, CO: Libraries Unlimited, Inc.
Ellis, A. (1993). The advantages and disadvantages of self-help therapy materials. *Professional Psychology, Research and Practice,* 24; 335-339.
Homme, L. E. (1965). Perspectives in psychology, XXIV: Control of coverants, the operants of the mind. *Psychological Record,* 15; 501-511.
Johnson, D. W., and Johnson, R. (1975). *Learning together and alone: Cooperation, competition, and individualization.* Englewood Cliffs, NJ: Prentice-Hall.
Johnson, D. W. and Johnson, R. (1981). *Reaching out: Interpersonal effectiveness and self-actualization,* second edition. Englewood Cliffs, NJ: Prentice-Hall.
Orton, G. L. (1997). *Strategies for counseling with children and their parents.* Pacific Grove, CA: Brooks/Cole Publishing.

Pardeck, J. T. (1992). Using bibliotherapy in treatment with children in residential care. *Residential Treatment for Children and Youth,* 9; 73-90.

Pardeck, J. T. (1993). *Using bibliotherapy in clinical practice: A guide to self-help books.* Westport, CT: Greenwood Press.

Pardeck, J. T. (1996). *Social work practice: An ecological approach.* Westport, CT: Auburn House.

Pardeck, J. T., and Pardeck, J. A. (1987). Using bibliotherapy to help children cope with the changing family. *Social Work in Education,* 9; 107-116.

Pardeck, J. T., and Pardeck, J. A. (1989). Bibliotherapy: A tool for helping preschool children deal with developmental change related to family relationships. *Early Child Development and Care,* 47; 107-129.

Quackenbush, R. L. (1991). The prescription of self-help books by psychologists: A bibliography of selected bibliotherapy resources. *Psychotherapy,* 28; 671-677.

Riordan, R. J. (1991). Bibliotherapy revisited. *Psychological Reports,* 68; 306.

Rogers, C. (1969). *Freedom to learn.* Columbus, OH: Charles E. Merrill.

Santrock, J. W., Minnett, A. M., and Campbell, B. D. (1994). *The authoritative guide to self-help books.* New York: The Guilford Press.

Skinner, B. F. (1953). *Science and human behavior.* New York: The Free Press.

Starker, S. (1988). Psychologists and self-help books: Attitudes and prescriptive practices of clinicians. *American Journal of Psychotherapy,* 42; 448-455.

Thompson, C. L., and Rudolph, L. B. (1996). *Counseling children,* fourth edition. Pacific Grove, CA: Brooks/Cole Publishing.

Wang, M., and Walberg, H. eds. (1985). *Adapting instruction to individual differences.* Berkeley, CA: McCutchan.

Chapter 3

Brown, L., and Brown, M. (1986). *Dinosaurs divorce: A guide for changing families.* Boston: Little, Brown.

Coleman, V. E. (1994). Lesbian battering: The relationship between personality and the perpetuation of violence. *Violence and Victims,* 9; 139-152.

DuBois, B., and Miley, K. K. (1996). *Social work: An empowering profession,* second edition. Needham Heights, MA: Allyn and Bacon.

Duncan, S. F., and Brown, G. (1992). RENEW: A program for building remarried family strengths. *Families in Society,* 73; 149-158.

Dutton, D. G. (1994). Patriarchy and wife assault: The ecological fallacy. *Violence and Victims,* 9; 167-182

Gardner, R. (1977). *The parents' book about divorce.* New York: Doubleday.

Gardner, R. (1983). *The boys' and girls' book about divorce.* Northvale, NJ: Jason Aronson.

Gardner, R. (1984). Counseling children in stepfamilies. *Elementary School Guidance and Counseling,* 19; 40-49.

Giblin, P. (1989). Use of reading assignments in clinical practice. *The American Journal of Family Therapy,* 17; 219-228.

Gladding, S. T. (1995). *Family therapy: History, theory, and practice.* Englewood Cliffs, NJ: Prentice-Hall, Inc.

Hartman, A. (1994). Diagrammatic assessment of family relationships. In B. R. Compton and B. Galaway (Eds.), *Social Work Processes,* fifth edition. Pacific Grove, CA: Brooks/Cole Publishing Company; 153-165.

Hepworth, D. H., Rooney, R. H., and Larsen, J. A. (1997). *Direct social work practice: Theory and skills,* fifth edition. Pacific Grove, CA: Brooks/Cole Publishing Company.

Jung, C. (1954). *Collected works: Psychology and alchemy.* New York: Pantheon Press.

Kalter, N. (1970). *Growing up with divorce.* New York: Free Press.

Kelly, P. (1992). Healthy step family functioning. *Families in Society,* 72; 579-587.

Kilpatrick, A. C., and Holland, T. P. (1995). *Working with families: An integrative model by level of functioning.* Needham Heights, MA: Allyn and Bacon.

Krementz, J. (1984). *How it feels when parents divorce.* New York: Knopf.

Marino, T. W. (1994). O. J. aftermath: The battering of American women. *Guidepost,* 37; 12, 23.

Maslow, A. (1971). *The farther reaches of human nature.* New York: Viking.

Melina, L. R. (1989). *Making sense of adoption.* New York: HarperCollins, Publishers, Inc.

Minuchin, S., and Nichols, M. (1993). *Family healing: Tales of hope and renewal from family therapy.* New York: The Free Press.

National Research Council. (1993). *Understanding child abuse and neglect.* Washington, DC: Author.

Orton, G. L. (1997). *Strategies for counseling with children and their parents.* Pacific Grove, CA: Brooks/Cole Publishing.

Papalia, D. E., and Olds, S. W. (1996). *A child's world: Infancy through adolescence,* seventh edition. New York: McGraw-Hill.

Pardeck, J. A., and Pardeck, J. T. (1986). *Books for early childhood: A developmental perspective.* Westport, CT: Greenwood Press.

Pardeck, J. T. (1990). An analysis of the deep structure preventing the development of a national policy for children and families in the United States. *Early Child Development and Care,* 57; 23-30.

Pardeck, J. T. (1993). *Using bibliotherapy in clinical practice: A guide to self-help books.* Westport, CT: Greenwood Press.

Pardeck, J. T. (1996). *Social work practice: An ecological approach.* Westport, CT: Auburn House.

Pardeck, J. T., and Yven, F. (1997). A family health approach to social work practice. *Family Therapy,* 24; 115-128.

Rubin, R. J. (1978). *A guide to theory and practice.* Phoenix, AZ: Oryx Press.

Rudman, M. K., Gagne, K. D., and Berstein, S. E. (1993). *Books to help children cope with separation and loss: An annotated bibliography,* fourth edition. New Providence, NJ: R. R. Bowker.

Schor, J. (1992). *The overworked American.* New York: Basic Books.

Seuling, B. (1985). *What kind of family is this?* Racine, WI: Western Publishing.
Starker, S. (1988). Psychologists and self-help books: Attitudes and prescriptive practices of clinicians. *American Journal of Psychotherapy,* 42; 448-455.
Thompson, C. L., and Rudolph, L. B. (1996). *Counseling children,* fourth edition. Pacific Grove, CA: Brooks/Cole Publishing.
Vega, W. A., and Murphy, J. W. (1990). *Culture and the restructuring of community mental health.* Westport, CT: Greenwood Press.
Walker, L. E. (1989). *Terrifying love: Why battered women kill and how society responds.* New York: Harper and Row.
Wallerstein, J., and Blakeslee, S. (1989). *Second chances.* New York: Ticknor and Fields.
Whitsett, D., and Land, H. (1992a). Role strain, coping, and marital satisfaction of stepparents. *Families in Society,* 73; 79-92.
Whitsett, D., and Land, H. (1992b). The development of a role strain index for stepparents. *Families in Society,* 73; 14-22
Wilson, J., and Blocher, L. (1990). The counselor's role in assisting children of alcoholics. *Elementary School Guidance and Counseling,* 25; 98-106.
Zaccaria, J., and Moses, H. (1968). *Facilitating human development through reading: The use of bibliotherapy in teaching and counseling.* Champaign, IL: Stipes.

Chapter 5

Bernstein, J. (1989). Bibliotherapy: How books can help children cope. In M. Rudman (Ed.), *Children's literature: Resource for the classroom.* New York: Christopher Gordon; 159-173.
Ellis, A. (1995). *Better, deeper, and more enduring brief therapy: The rational emotive behavior therapy approach.* New York: Brunner/Mazel Publishers.
Pardeck, J. T. (1994). Self-help books get mixed reviews. *The Psychotherapy Letter,* 6; 9.
Popple, P. R., and Leighninger, L. C. (1996). *Social work, social welfare, and American society.* Boston: Allyn and Bacon.
Santrock, J. W., Minnett, A. M., and Campbell, B. D. (1994). *The authoritative guide to self-help books.* New York: The Guilford Press.
Starker, S. (1988). Psychologists and self-help books: Attitudes and prescriptive practices of clinicians. *American Journal of Psychotherapy,* 42; 448-455.

Author Index

Includes authors and joint authors. Numbers refer to individual book entries in Chapter 4.

Title Index

Numbers refer to individual book entries in Chapter 4.

Subject Index

Numbers refer to individual book entries in Chapter 4.

Order Your Own Copy of This Important Book for Your Personal Library!

USING BOOKS IN CLINICAL SOCIAL WORK PRACTICE
A Guide to Bibliotherapy

_______ in hardbound at $29.95 (ISBN: 0-7890-0120-9)

_______ in softbound at $19.95 (ISBN: 0-7890-0430-5)

COST OF BOOKS _______

OUTSIDE USA/CANADA/ MEXICO: ADD 20% _______

POSTAGE & HANDLING _______
(US: $3.00 for first book & $1.25 for each additional book)
Outside US: $4.75 for first book & $1.75 for each additional book)

SUBTOTAL _______

IN CANADA: ADD 7% GST _______

STATE TAX _______
(NY, OH & MN residents, please add appropriate local sales tax)

FINAL TOTAL _______
(If paying in Canadian funds, convert using the current exchange rate. UNESCO coupons welcome.)

☐ **BILL ME LATER:** ($5 service charge will be added)
(Bill-me option is good on US/Canada/Mexico orders only; not good to jobbers, wholesalers, or subscription agencies.)

☐ Check here if billing address is different from shipping address and attach purchase order and billing address information.

Signature _______________

☐ **PAYMENT ENCLOSED:** $ _______________

☐ **PLEASE CHARGE TO MY CREDIT CARD.**

☐ Visa ☐ MasterCard ☐ AmEx ☐ Discover
☐ Diners Club
Account # _______________

Exp. Date _______________

Signature _______________

Prices in US dollars and subject to change without notice.

NAME _______________

INSTITUTION _______________

ADDRESS _______________

CITY _______________

STATE/ZIP _______________

COUNTRY _______________ COUNTY (NY residents only) _______________

TEL _______________ FAX _______________

E-MAIL _______________
May we use your e-mail address for confirmations and other types of information? ☐ Yes ☐ No

Order From Your Local Bookstore or Directly From

The Haworth Press, Inc.

10 Alice Street, Binghamton, New York 13904-1580 • USA
TELEPHONE: 1-800-HAWORTH (1-800-429-6784) / Outside US/Canada: (607) 722-5857
FAX: 1-800-895-0582 / Outside US/Canada: (607) 772-6362
E-mail: getinfo@haworth.com

PLEASE PHOTOCOPY THIS FORM FOR YOUR PERSONAL USE.

BOF96